States of Exile

States of Exile

*Correspondences Between
Art, Literature,
and Nursing*

Jeanine Young-Mason

National League for Nursing Press • *New York*
Pub. No. 14-2632

The cover photograph, a detail of "The Burghers of Calais," and all interior photographs of "The Burghers of Calais" are by the author.

ISBN 0-88737-626-6

This book was set in Janson by Publications Development Company, Crockett,
Texas. The editor and designer was Allan Graubard. The printer was Clarkwood
Corp. The cover was designed by Lauren Stevens.

Printed in the United States of America.

Dedicated

to

my parents

Harold and Catherine Young

About the Author

Commitment to nursing's philosophical and pragmatic ideals embodies Professor Young-Mason's teaching, research, consultation, and writing. Her work on the development of the concept of compassion has been published in the nursing literature and other scholarly periodicals. Her primary sources for this thematic research are literature, fine art, film, and published personal narratives of psychiatric and somatic illness. Young-Mason's research has taken her to Japan, France, Ireland, England, Scotland, Iraq, and Morocco. One particular project, a video film "Visual Clues to Emotional States," was filmed in France at Rodin's last home and studio.

Dr. Young-Mason's regular column, "Nursing and the Arts," in *Clinical Nurse Specialist: The Journal for Advanced Nursing Practice*, highlights the ways in which art and literature enrich and instruct nursing practice. She is author of *21 Words for Nurses* (Diamond Press, 1995) a book for meditation on words relevant to nurses.

Young-Mason joined the faculty of the School of Nursing at the University of Massachusetts at Amherst in 1985 from Massachusetts General Hospital where she was a clinical nurse specialist on the consultation-liaison nursing service. A graduate of the University of Michigan School of Nursing, she holds a Master's Degree in Psychiatric-Mental Health Nursing from Boston University School of Nursing and a Doctoral Degree from Boston University in Humanistic and Behavioral Studies. Her research has been funded by the University, Sigma Theta Tau International Honor Society in Nursing, and the Kittredge Foundation.

Jeanine Young-Mason, Ed.D., R.N., C.S., Associate Professor, is a Fellow of the American Academy of Nursing.

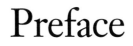

Preface

A humanities education can give nurses the tools to cope with the pain, helplessness, loneliness, joy and relief, and the day-to-day grind encountered in the world of the health vulnerable. It must be one of the main tasks of nursing curricula to teach the use of these tools.

Em Olivia Bevis, 1993

This text is intended as a contribution to the development of compassionate nurses. It aims to provide student nurses and their teachers with a fuller knowledge of the nature of suffering and the need for compassion, specifically demonstrating the ways in which values, beliefs, perceptions, and spirituality affect behavior, health, and healing. Our common heritage of the healing arts—painting, sculpture, film, and literature—can heal morally, spiritually, and ultimately, physically, those who suffer from illness and ignorance. The healing arts accomplish this through evocation, depiction, entertainment, and wisdom.

Each chapter can be considered a study for a class seminar of a semester-length course in reading, writing, and reasoning in nursing studies. It incorporates selected works of art and literature as primary sources for this study. These works afford students studying the human condition with a modality by which they can consider the correspondences between art and nursing phenomena. It also encourages the full expression of thought, concern, and development of reasoning in discussion and writing. This enhancement of students' understanding fosters an articulation of personal perceptions and values and a recognition and appreciation of others. The experience of studying depictions of the vicissitudes of the human condition in the classroom clarifies and deepens, thus fortifying students for the actual clinical experiences which so often perplex, mystify, and distress. This crucial undertaking is also meant to counterbalance the prevalent scientific and technologic aspects of nursing education.

Each chapter begins with a précis of a work of art or literature. Selected passages, examples of art, and photographs are cited to illustrate specific subjects for discussion. These excerpts and photographs are then discussed by students in their own words. Following each discussion student stories which were written in response to a theme drawn from the art or literary work are included.

The works of art and literature were chosen, in part, due to their inherent dialectic which stimulates students' sense of argument and analogy to everyday life and its contentions, oppositions, and polarizations.

The concluding section provides a working definition of compassion drawn from the exploration of the art, film, and literature presented in this text. The remarks in Notes to Students and Teachers are meant to invite and to encourage nurse educators and their students to delve into this study. It explains why it is imperative that this work within the nursing curricula be conducted by nurse educators. The methodology of the author is included here as are essay questions based upon the selected works within this text. Finally, other works of art, film, and literature utilized for this study are listed with full citation, according to major themes.

Throughout the text the designation SN stands for Student Nurse. As the class discussions progress, works studied in previous chapters are mentioned as analogies are made.

- *Chapter One, The Exile of Sacrifice: Rodin, "The Burghers of Calais."* The Burghers were six men who offered their lives as a sacrifice to save the starving citizens of the besieged city of Calais during the 100 Years War. In Rodin's sculptural masterpiece, the human portrayal of suffering and sacrifice becomes universal evoking correspondence between the contemporary viewer and these secular martyrs of 1347.

- *Chapter Two, The Exile of Passivity: Kurosawa, Ikiru.* Ikiru translates to "to live" and tells of a middle aged Japanese man and Chief of the Citizen's Bureau whose dull, monotonous routine as a petty official has deadened him to life. When he learns of his stomach cancer and impending death, he suddenly questions why he has been living at all. As he bravely searches for a way to give his life meaning he becomes revitalized.

- *Chapter Three, The Exile of Abandonment: Sophocles, Philoktetes. Philoktetes* is a legend about a soldier who is banished by his society because of his troublesome behavior. He has a wound that will not heal and his unceasing cries and complaints are intolerable. However, when Philoktetes' possession, Achilles' magical bow, is needed by this same society to fight the Trojan War, all concerned must contend with bitterness and deception.

- *Chapter Four, The Exile of Illness: Tolstoi, The Death of Ivan Ilych.* Ivan Ilych is the story of a lawyer and magistrate in 19th century Russia whose last illness separates him from his family, friends, and doctors. In this middle class society none can transcend their self protective, superficial existence in order to recognize fully Ivan's plight. Ivan's spiritual journey in the form of an inner dialogue is recorded in intimate detail.

- *Chapter Five, The Exile of Emotional Disorder: Bernanos, Mouchette, and Cather, "Paul's Case."* Mouchette is a poor, 14-year-old French girl who lives in a small French village. Her tenacious, defiant nature allows her to survive all manner of insults from classmates and villagers until she is deceived and raped by a friend of her father's. Paul is a teenage boy who attends Pittsburgh High School. He is a theatrical young man given to day dreaming. In fact, he needs his fantasy life in order to tolerate the day-to-day existence of home and school. But it is the fantasy life which his teachers and father inadvertently crush. When both teenagers are robbed of defiance and dreams, their very modes of survival in their stark worlds, they cannot find a way to cling to life.

- *Chapter Six, The Exile of Grief: Mason, Gilgamesh. Gilgamesh* is an ancient legend about a king who lost a friend to death who after a long time of grief turned his life into a journey to find eternal life, or failing that, to come to terms with his own mortality.

- The *Conclusion* treats of a full definition of compassion derived from the works of art and literature explored in this textbook.

- *Notes to Students and Teachers* invites students and their teachers to undertake the exploration of the correspondences between art and literature and nursing phenomena for enrichment and understanding. It provides methodological questions designed for this work. Finally, it includes essay questions, based upon the art, film, and literature presented in this text to further assist students of the human condition.

- The *Bibliography* provides the sources for the works of art, literature, and film cited within this textbook.

- *Appendix A* provides a selection of works of art, film, and literature which have been studied employing this same methodology. They are arranged according to major themes of: beginning nursing practice; character studies; and the roots of poverty and disease.

- *Appendix B* provides the reader with the full citations for the footnotes found within the essay in Chapter One on "The Burghers of Calais."

Contents

The Exile of Sacrifice: Rodin, "The Burghers of Calais"

Sadly, in difficult times we tend to shrug off the spiritual heritage of artists from an 'easier age' with 'What use is that sort of thing to us now?' It is an understandable but short-sighted reaction. And utterly impoverishing. [Artists] should be willing to act as balm for all wounds.

Etty Hillesum

RODIN, "THE BURGHERS OF CALAIS"

"Pierre-Auguste Rodin was commissioned in 1884 by the Municipal Council of Calais, France, to design a monument to honor the secular martyrdom of the Burghers of Calais. These six men had offered their lives as a sacrifice in 1347 to end the eleven-month siege of Calais by King Edward III of England during the Hundred Years

---

Portions of the précis appeared in the *Journal of Professional Nursing* and presentations given at the Hirshhorn Museum and Sculpture Garden, Smithsonian Institution, Washington, D.C. for the Society for Health and Human Values and the Museum of Fine Arts in Springfield, Massachusetts for the Eldering Consortium on Aging and the Humanities.

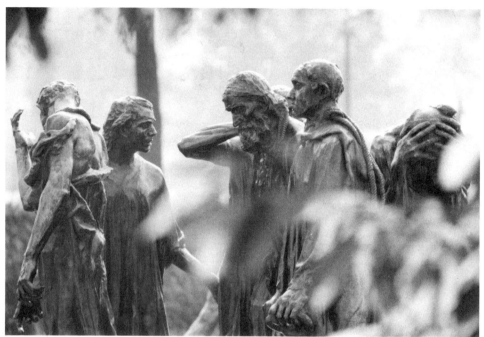

Burghers of Calais, bronze, 1884.

In the well-known, recorded Gsell-Rodin conversations of 1911, Gsell summarized Rodin's theory of the expressiveness of the human image: "Generally the face alone is considered to be the mirror of the soul: the mobility of the features of the face seems to us the unique exteriorization of the spiritual life. In reality, there is not one muscle of the body that does not express variations within. Each speaks of joy or sadness, enthusiasm or despair, calm or rage. Outstretched arms, an unrestrained torso can smile with as much sweetness as eyes or lips. But in order to be able to interpret all aspects of the flesh, one must be trained patiently in the spelling and reading of this beautiful book." (*Art: Conversations with Paul Gsell.* Translated by deCaso J., Sanders P.B. Berkeley, CA University of California Press, 1984, p. 10.) The question thus arises, how can we, as students of the human condition, undertake this necessary training? How might we develop the aesthetic senses to appreciate the legibility of the human face and form more fully? For assistance in this undertaking we naturally turn to the artist. For the artist "sees" the world through eyes trained to acutely appreciate color, light and shadow, surface and volume, and inner truth. In particular, the education and training of Rodin, and the development of his artistic technique and insight, offer the health care professional rich intellectual material for this study. A closer look at Rodin's masterpiece, "The Burghers of Calais," amply illustrates this vision. (Young-Mason, 1990, p. 289)

War. This event was vividly described by Froissart in his *Chronicles*. The *Chronicles* documented the events of this day, recounting the desperate state of the starving citizens of Calais. Even the names of the Burghers are available to us." (Young-Mason, 1990, p. 289)

"This period in medieval history had been a favorite of Rodin's. Once awarded the commission, he began work on the piece by studying the *Chronicles* and visiting the site of this historical event. He searched among his own contemporaries for models for the monument who would be of the ethnic type of Calais' citizens and who would represent ordinary men. Rodin fashioned six separate identities whose physiognomies reflected states of soul uniquely distinct from one another. It is of interest to note that an English priest of about this same period of history (14th Century) described the faculties of the soul as 'the three major ones of Mind which includes Memory, Reason, and Will, and two minor ones, Imagination and Sensuality."[3]

Rodin's method of capturing these states of soul was unusual. He first modeled his figures nude, making small, quick "sketches" in clay to capture what he called "fugitive truth." His premise was that these quick sketches of the model caught the exteriorization of inner truths more accurately than working deliberately from the posed, stationary model.[4] "This method enabled him to decipher the expressions of feelings in all parts of the body."[5] He draped the figures only after he was satisfied that their physiognomies expressed full representation of an inner psychological state. Geoffroy, an art critic and contemporary of Rodin's, stated after viewing the first three figures completed that "they were not mere depictions, but each (had) a corporeal presence, like that of a living person."[5] The artist began the nudes and

> before he even thought about the arrangement of the draperies, he placed beneath them skeletons, nervous systems, and all the organs of life and of creatures of flesh and blood. . . . They also represent man's ephemeral existence and his sorrows. They bear the mark of sadness which is the unavoidable characteristic of all great works. (Young-Mason, 1990, p. 290)

"Numerous scholars have painstakingly analyzed the work for clues to Rodin's artistic and literary inspiration for the Burghers.[2]

One thought is that he chose not the abstract emotion of devotion, but a specific episode from the Froissart narrative, the departure of the Burghers to the camp of Edward III.[6] (He selected) the crucial moment just after the six men volunteered to sacrifice their lives in order to save their besieged city."[2] The King, whose intention was to humiliate these brave men, had ordered that they strip to their chemises, place the rope by which they were to be hanged around their necks, and, bearing the keys to the city gate and Citadel, walk barefoot to his camp to meet their fate.[1] These men were to be King Edward's trophies of war to compensate him for losses of men and money during the eleven-month siege.

Rainier Maria Rilke, the celebrated poet who was Rodin's secretary for three years, "felt that the monument was not an attempt to re-create an episode from the Hundred Years War, but an attempt to use that episode to make a statement on the meaning of life and death."[2] Elsen, the noted Rodin scholar, suggests that Rodin wished the Burghers to be read like a six-act play, a succession of movements and emotions, in a composition like a chaplet, a living rosary."[2] McNamara, another Rodin scholar, holds that ultimately the Burghers represent the various emotional states that all pass through when they learn that they are going to die.[2] These conclusions are based in large part on Rodin's own comments to Paul Gsell, a French writer and his contemporary, that he wanted the Burghers to be seen "like a living rosary of suffering and sacrifice."[1]

It is this view of the Burghers—that they form a chaplet, a living rosary—that seems best to describe the interplay of emotions and reflections evoked by the work as a whole. For as one approaches these large figures standing silently in the garden of the Musée Rodin in Paris, or the gardens of Parliament in London, the viewer is drawn singly to each particular figure in succession. It is my supposition that each figure in some way represents a communion with the viewer's state of soul at that moment. After entering into this private communication with one Burgher, the spectator is slowly pulled towards the next, and then the next. It is not until one has circled the figures completely that one realizes that these six separate men also represent the emotions of human beings facing death.

Rodin once claimed that his wish was that the Burghers would represent a communion between the living and the dead.[7] And is this not what this chaplet truly is? Emotions, recollected scenes, gestures, and faces flood the mind of the reflective viewer of these symbols of humanity. These powerful representations of the complex states of sorrow, fear, resignation, quiet rage, and disbelief stir memories of interactions not quite understood, behaviors unexplained, personal losses endured, and sacrifices made on behalf of others. It may be at once comforting and disquieting to the spectator to be reminded that these bewildering moments are common to humanity throughout time." (Young-Mason, 1990, p. 291)

CLASS DISCUSSION

After hearing the story of the conception and evolution of "The Burghers of Calais," students were shown the photographic slides of the sculpture. They were then asked "Does this sculpture evoke memories of scenes or gestures of individuals known to you in your personal or professional life? Please describe your scene and your understanding of its meaning. Did the depiction of the Burghers change or influence your view of this incident in any way? If so, how?

STUDENTS' MEDITATIONS ON THE BURGHERS

Ideally, students would be able to view the Burghers of Calais directly. This would be possible in Philadelphia, Los Angeles, and also in Paris, Brussels, Basel, Copenhagen and Tokyo. However, it is still possible to accomplish this work in the classroom of the student nurse through the utilization of good quality photographs, as illustrated here. These recorded meditations were written in the classroom by students introduced to the above material who then viewed the photographs reprinted here.

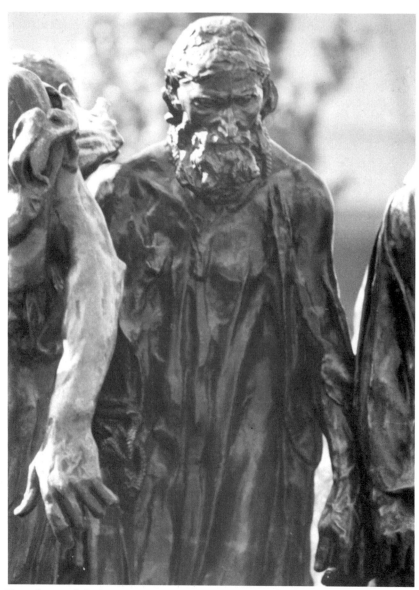

Burghers of Calais, detail.

The six men are bound together not only visually by the rope, but spiritually by their common purpose. Their common offer of self-sacrifice was initiated by Eustache de St. Pierre, the oldest and richest of the Burghers, who stands at the forefront of the cortège. His aging, emaciated body is visible beneath his thin garment. His long beard does not hide his gaunt cheeks; his eyes are sunken in his forehead and they look far off beyond the spectator. His long arms, gnarled with veins, hang limply at his sides. He said to his fellow citizens on hearing the King's decree on that fateful day, "Sir, it would be a cruel and miserable thing to allow such a population to die, so long as some remedy can be found. To prevent such a misfortune would surely be an act of great merit in our Saviour's eyes and, for my part, I should have strong hopes of receiving pardon for my sins if I died to save this people and thus I wish to be the first to come forward. I am willing to strip to my shirt, bare my head, put the rope around my neck, and deliver myself to the King of England's camp."[1] He walks with resignation, in quiet submission. (Young-Mason, 1990, p. 293)

Eustache de St. Pierre

The passage of time and troubles has brought about an image of emaciation and dejection, the eyes and body language evoke a memory from my childhood that will never be forgotten. Standing beside the apple tree that summer, I see my grand father leaning on his rake, head down, eyes focused on the ground, staring blankly. My grandfather's expression was similar to that of Eustache de St. Pierre . . . a look of uncertainty, perhaps fearing what the future held. This sculpture of Eustache de St. Pierre has evoked a feeling of understanding and closeness for my grandfather that I never felt while he was alive.

Mark Richardson

I think that of all the figures in Rodin's "Burghers of Calais," the one that stands out most is the old man, Eustache de St. Pierre. His appearance saddens me greatly. He looks as if he has resigned himself to his death. For such a strong man, of such honor and integrity to be so submissive is a sight, and most certainly emotion, that pulls heart strings. I am reminded of older men who have lived healthy, active lives and are suddenly struck by an illness that will forever change their futures. It is an emotion of hopelessness—"this is the end and I must submit to whatever is to be." The sad, yet determined look in this man's face and his stooped posture compliment and contradict each other. He is trying to show his strength as a man by doing what he feels he must. However, his stooped posture clues the viewer into the fact that he is walking slowly, perhaps reliving in his mind significant moments of his life. He has given up in body, but never in spirit.

Brenda Jones

When I view this sculpture, which I have never seen before, I can't help but be overwhelmed by the internal pain that they [the figures] so clearly express. I know that I have had experiences in my life which these men could remind me of, but I am completely unable to draw them from my memory. It seems that the incredible nobility of their story and situation would be lessened by my attempt at comparison.

Each one of these men, as portrayed by Rodin, is experiencing the same situation in a completely different way. But is it really the same situation? Each man has had different experience of life. Their perspectives on life in this world depend on many factors—but ultimately they do have to give up one common possession, their very lives.

Looking at the sculpture of Eustache de St. Pierre, the oldest and richest of the Burghers, I am particularly moved. Humility, nobility, sacrifice, love, hope and great faith—these are qualities that his character powerfully exudes. To be the first to step forward in any situation, no matter how great or small, requires courage. The courage this man possessed to sacrifice his life for the lives of others is truly amazing. And courage, as I mentioned before, is certainly not the only quality that enabled his action. Having thought about these things, and seeing his submissive acceptance which, as he was aware, was the only solution, someone similar comes to mind—Jesus Christ. I realize that this man was just that—a man—and it is not my intention to deify him. However, it is obvious that Eustache de St. Pierre was aware of the sacrifice that would please his creator and he certainly lived by his conviction.

Kerri O'Malley

I have seen Eustache de St. Pierre before. He is the frail, elderly gentleman sadly resigned to spending his last years in a nursing home. He walks just like this man with downcast eyes that look beyond events going on around him. He is a proud man who enjoyed his own home, woodworking, gardening, entertaining friends and family. Now he is on Medicaid, his home is gone, his woodworking tools have been sold, his fishing gear given away. His sole possession is his recliner chair and his undaunted spirit and wit that eases his visitors.

J. H. Kay

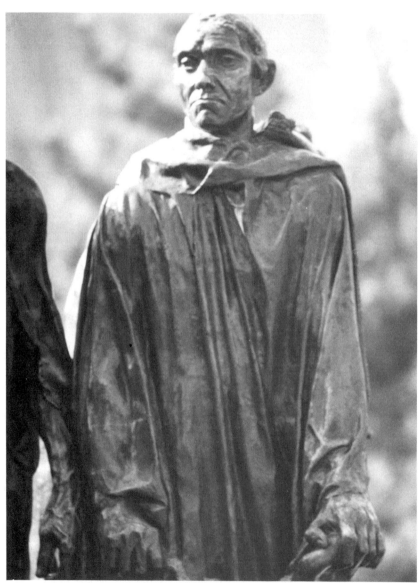

Burghers of Calais, detail.

Following him, Jean d'Aire, another greatly respected and wealthy citizen, stood up and said that he would go with his friend.[1] This man, younger than the first, stands stalwart, his body rigid with anger. He has much to lose—his life is half lived and he will never see his two daughters mature. His hands fiercely clench the key to the city. His eyes glare above his grimly set mouth and furrowed brow. Deep hollows along his jaw line and cheeks tell of his city's starvation. The unjustness of this humiliating sacrifice is too much to bear, but bear it he is determined to do. (Rodin modeled Jean d'Aire after his only son.) (Young-Mason, 1990, p. 294)

Jean d'Aire

Jean d'Aire powerfully reminds me of my own feelings of the despair in this world. I always felt I was put on this earth to make a significant change. In Jean d'Aire's time, the King was unjust in forcing these men to their death, for no crime was committed. His power and control reminds me of our government officials today. Of course, it is a little different; however, many officials are responsible for injustice and neglect. Jean d'Aire's eyes filled with pity, frustration and disgust—I identify with him. I feel unable to make a difference. I used to feel hope, now just frustration and fear. The selfishness of King Edward seems to have been passed down to our government officials. I often grit my teeth in anger that I can barely control. I see this, also, in Jean d'Aire.

What I am trying to say is that my goal is to significantly change the way society thinks and judges. I want to convince others not to judge but to treat everyone with the respect and dignity we all deserve. The nursing homes of today take respect and dignity away from the elderly. I want to give it back.

Anonymous

Jean d'Aire reminds me of a picture that I saw in the *Boston Globe*. It was the face of one young man, the brother of a slain police detective. The photograph was taken after a court proceeding in which a judge dismissed all charges against the man who had been arrested for killing his brother. The judge had ruled that the man would not receive a fair trial because the police intentionally failed to produce an informant whose testimony might have cleared the accused. The face of this young brother, upon hearing this, resembles Jean d'Aire in remarkable ways. You can see the intense anger in the set jaw, the sense of despair that he must have been feeling gives his eyes a particularly heavy, brooding look. And the way that his mouth was turned down at the corners, all of that was in this photograph. To me, his sense of betrayal is very evident. It seems that there are some parallels in what happened to this brother of the detective and Jean d'Aire. Though Jean d'Aire is giving up his life, and this is the ultimate sacrifice, this man will never be able to see his brother's accused murderer brought to justice. His loss is two-fold: he mourns his brother and he is betrayed by the system that his brother lost his life for. His life is forever changed.

Anonymous

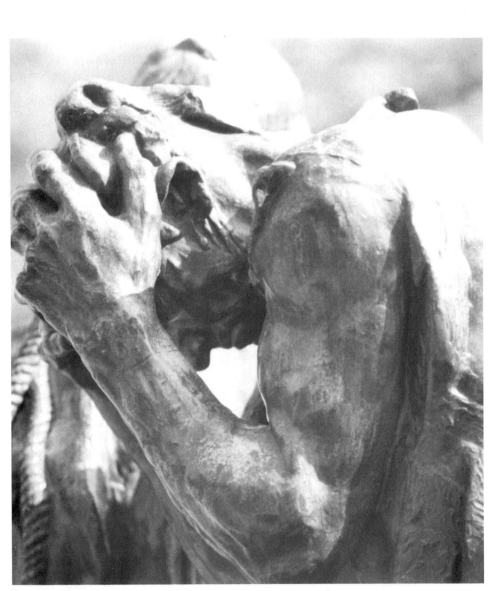

Burghers of Calais, detail.

Directly behind Jean d'Aire, a man with bowed shoulders faces away from the others. His large hands and arms press heavily against his head and body. Andrieus d'Andres, one of the two men whose names were discovered in the Vatican archives, is consumed with grief that he cannot master. He holds himself in with such force that his arm and chest muscles bulge from the effort. He has shielded his face in this gesture so completely that the spectator's gaze seems an intrusion. (Young-Mason, p. 295)

Andrieus d'Andres

Caring for older adults in their homes, I have on many occasions been witness to despair. Despair brought on by illness, depression, dementia, social or economic circumstances. Andrieus d'Andres personifies the hopelessness that these individuals feel. They are beyond reaching out, beyond prayer, beyond communication except with themselves. There is a pulling inward away from the reality of deep hurt. It reminds me of those who return to the fetal position.

Anonymous

Andrieus d'Andres "consumed with grief that he cannot master . . . holds himself in with such force that his arm and chest muscles bulge from the effort" (Young-Mason, 1994, p. 295) reminds me of a patient that I care for twice a week. Three weeks ago she was diagnosed with a rare form of cancer and told that she had 3 to 4 years left to live. She no sooner heard the word "cancer" when she was handed a pamphlet on colostomy care and then sent home with the words "try not to worry."

Yesterday, as I sat with her, she broke down sobbing. She concealed her face the same way as Andrieus d'Andres and mumbled "I am not supposed to cry, but I have to get it out somehow." The man in this sculpture and this woman are experiencing similar strong emotions, death lies ahead and the fear overwhelms their entire being, physically and emotionally.

Jennifer Cashman

Andrieus d'Andres is so stricken by grief that he cannot look up, but instead encloses himself in to a sort of physical barrier from the world. He brings back memories of a burial of a friend of mine who died unexpectedly one month after high school graduation. At the grave site, his mother expressed her grief similarly. I had never before, or since, witnessed such incredible pain. She enclosed her head with her hands as if to say to the world . . . "You could never understand the hurt I am feeling."

Kristy MacNaughton

Andrieus d'Andres is the man who holds his head in his hands consumed with grief. This man and his position of sorrow immediately called to my mind a scene which occurred a few years ago. I walked into my parent's bedroom and found my father sitting with his head in his hands, much like the man in this sculpture. He had just learned that his father had died and he was beside himself. It was the one and only time I have ever seen my father cry or exhibit such an intense emotional state.

Amy Klausmayer

The man, Andrieus d'Andres, brings to mind a very vivid image for me. When I was a freshman in high school one of my classmates committed suicide. The news hit the school late on the day of her death, after school hours. By the next morning everyone had heard. When the day started the school was in chaos. My classmates, for the most part, didn't attend classes that day. They spent it roaming the halls in turmoil. At one point an assembly was called. I can picture people from that day who resemble each of the Burghers, but most striking is a young man named Mike.

Mike sat front and center of the auditorium with his feet on the chair in front of him, his elbows on his knees and his head in his hands. His fingers gripped his hair. He had physically made himself into an impenetrable box. He was surrounded by people on all sides. They were trying to touch him, to talk to him; to reach him. But he was literally a brick. Every muscle in his body was clenched. He looked inward, he saw no one else. At times he wept openly, hysterically. At the end of the assembly, the room emptied but he just sat, immobile, screaming. The people around him had pulled back and no longer tried to penetrate his awareness. They just sat staring blankly at him and each other. Eventually he was alone in the room. I don't think he noticed. When I look at the picture of Andrieus d'Andres I hear Mike's screams.

Danielle Pierotti

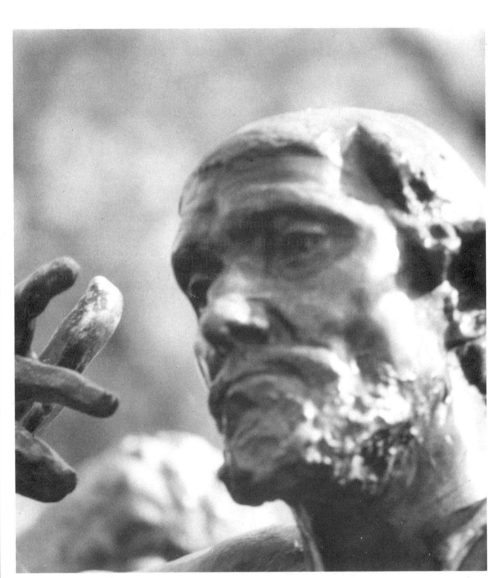

Burghers of Calais, detail.

Behind Andrieus d'Andres is Jacques d'Weissant, the third man to proffer his life. He, too, owned a rich family estate.[1] His face is an echo of Jean d'Aire's. His eyes gaze beyond the spectator and his companions, lost in private thoughts. His right arm raised with fingers spread, he appears to stumble forward, caught midway between saying good-bye and "listening for farewells."[6] (Young-Mason, 1990, p. 296)

Jacques d'Weissant

I grew up in a town settled mainly by French Canadians. The set of the jaw is very familiar. If you know French characteristics, these men express them all. The face of Jacques d'Weissant reminds me of an elderly man I observed in 1969. My husband's cousin had died of a brain tumor at age 25. The morning of the funeral, his grandfather came into the funeral parlor and looked at young Gerald in the same way. He looked beyond all of us, stumbling forward, leaning on his cane, saying his private "Good-bye."

Diane Murphy

I relate most to Jacques d'Weissant. I see determined resignation on his face. His jaw is clenched and his mouth pursed. He leans forward as if his thoughts and jaw lead him. He understands, intellectually, that his sacrifice must be made, his jaw outthrust in determination to carry this necessary evil through. His eyes are tired and slightly downcast in an accepting expression of resignation. His hand is thrust up half shielding him, as if it prevents him from looking too far forward to his inevitable end. The falling, stumbling gait is, despite his mindful decision, because the body fails; succumbing to the jelly knees and fainting feeling that comes with sheer terror. Jacques d'Weissant is stronger than his body. He has left his body, he is living through his reason, his intellect, and his determination. I see him as a man morally motivated, having achieved a high level of self-actualization. He is willing to commit to self-sacrifice for the good of the whole. He understands that through his death others will have life. (He is probably a parent.)

Catherine McGarty

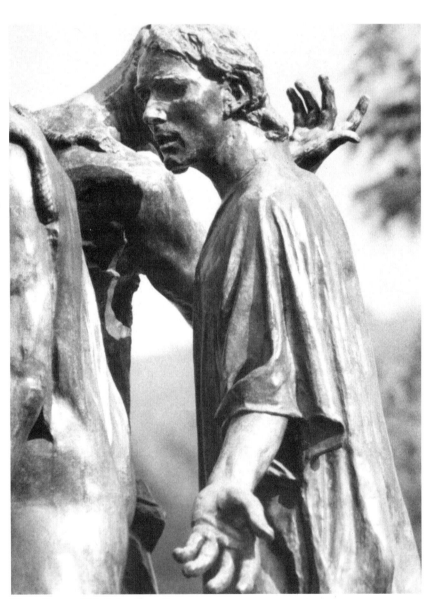

Burghers of Calais, detail.

◄ To the right of Andrieus d'Andres walks a youthful, handsome boy, not much more than a teenager. His name is Jean d'Fiennes. His appearance is so contemporary that it startles the viewer. This slim boy with smooth cheeks and choir-like robe cannot believe what is happening to him. His eyes are wide with incredulity and fear. His hands are thrown up with palms outward as though he is asking all those around him, "Why?" (Young-Mason, 1990, p. 297)

Jean d'Fiennes

The sculpture of Jean d'Fiennes brings back many personal memories and emotions. My mother passed away almost four years ago and this sculpture exemplifies the bewilderment and grief that I experienced. His expression and gestures remind me of how lost and confused I felt, as though it wasn't really happening. It is a numb feeling and very frightening; it seemed as if I had lost control over events in my life and wasn't sure what to feel or do.

The whole of the sculpture reminds me of my family and our reactions to my mother's death. We went through the next few days and weeks bound together by our grief yet each going through his or her own, very personal turmoil. I feel a great compassion for these men because, although the circumstances are very different, the emotions are the same.

Julie Amaral

Jean d'Fiennes, the youngest Burgher, reminds me of many adolescent boys I have known on an adolescent psychiatric unit. The gesture of the hands is especially evocative. They seem to ask "why is this happening, what has happened to put me here, in this place?" And some ask "why is it so hard to grow up?" The sculpture has not changed my view of these boys but it has universalized it.

Anonymous

Jean d'Fiennes looks remarkably like a friend of mine who just received the news that his father was hospitalized due to a stroke. When I saw my friend, his face was expressionless as if there were nothing there within. His shoulders were low as he leaned forward and stared at the ground. His hands hung out at his sides and it looked like he had no feelings, just emptiness. When he spoke his speech was slow and the tone of it was filled with disbelief. It was as if he did not know what happened to him or what to do.

Cathy Bamford

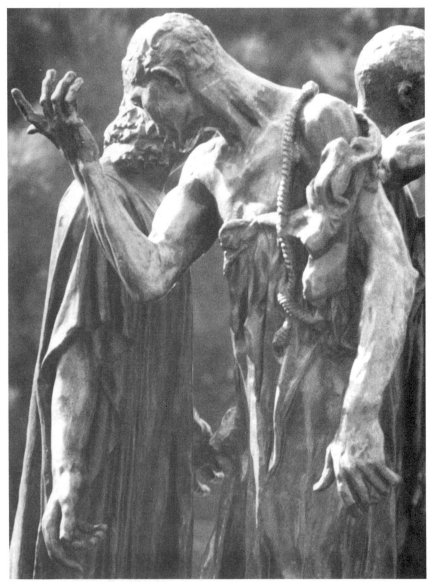

Burghers of Calais, detail.

The figure of young Pierre d'Weissant seems the most complicated—his torso and head are twisted to the right, his arm is raised up across his body shielding his face. It is apparent that he is weeping—nostrils flared, mouth agape, eyebrows tightly knitted. His disturbing, yet "vague gesture"[6] is complex. This premature death, which is so unnecessary, has overwhelmed him and he has lost control. The only solution to gaining composure is to turn inward—no one can help him forestall the inevitable. He is to give up his young life; hope has flown. (This man is the brother of Jacques d'Weissant, the third figure discussed.)[1] (Young-Mason, 1990, p. 298)

Pierre d'Weissant

Pierre d'Weissant's gesture—his arm raised across his body shielding his face and his apparent weeping—explain to me, finally, a disturbing event which occurred in a child psychiatric hospital many years ago. I had not understood my own action of that day until I saw this Burgher. His premature death has overwhelmed him and there seems to be no one to help. Hope has flown away.

I had been gaining clinical experience as a senior student nurse at this hospital. For several months I had spent a great deal of time with two adolescent boys, one had set fire to the family home on several occasions, the other had inadvertently stood by and watched his younger brother drown. It was felt that their specific disorders were not amenable to further treatment in their present setting. They would have to be transferred to the state psychiatric hospital. I had seen the state facility and was devastated that these two young boys were being sent there. It seemed like incarceration to me.

When the state attendants came for the second boy in the same week, my sense of discouragement deepened. I promised to accompany this boy down to the state van. As we approached the locked unit doors, he remembered his winter jacket left behind on his bed. I volunteered to retrieve it so as to save him having to make that walk to the door twice. After all, the rest of the kids on the unit knew that he was too sick to stay, and they knew where he was going. In a way, it felt as though everyone was giving up on these two boys. I worried about their pride and then I worried about the fear that the other children felt—this could happen to them. When I attempted to return to the child and the state attendants waiting by the locked doors, I was utterly unable to move toward them. Instead, I spontaneously threw the jacks into the air toward them with just such a gesture as Pierre d'Weissant's. Now I understand what that gesture meant . . . it seemed as though hope had flown away, no one could intervene. I could do nothing to prevent this boy's fate. I had to gain my composure for my own sake, and for the child's. Many people watched that day, but no one came forward. . . .

Anonymous

Pierre d'Weissant's open grief and shock immediately bring to mind the mother of my infant patient who was diagnosed as having a fatal degenerative neurological disease. When I met them the baby had just been admitted with "hypotonia" and during the two days I helped care for them it slowly became apparent to us all that the baby's condition was extremely serious and that she would not get well.

Although they said nothing at the time, the technicians in the myelogram room confirmed the mother's worst fears, that her child had inherited some type of awful disease. Throughout this dreadful day of test after test, the mother's face grew paler, her eyes took on a look of disbelief. She would hold her baby, stare at her for the longest time. She seemed very far away, lost in thought. Tears would suddenly swell up in her eyes as she looked out the window totally unaware of her environment.

By the second day when a muscle biopsy gave the final clinical diagnoses, the mother was distraught. She couldn't look at anyone, but would stand as if unable to bear what she might hear, her arms were often outstretched as if to say "why my baby?" Her lips were set in a determined line which she was often unable to hold because of her grief. At times she cried openly. I found her curled up in a chair at one point, staring off, tears streaming down her face. It is here that she reflects Pierre d'Weissant. When I approached her she lifted her arm and turned away from me, unable to comprehend her baby's future. She didn't seem to really see me but was totally isolated in her sorrow, lost in her private grief.

Adrienne Fleming

Pierre d'Weissant evokes a scene from the city hospital neurological unit that is always with me. This man looked like Pierre in many ways, but it is the response of both men to irretrievable loss that startles me. The man at city hospital was a college professor who had been shot in an attempted hold up on his way to teach an evening class. The gunshot wound to his temple did not interfere with his ability to think but it had paralyzed his whole right side. The afternoon of the second day of his admission he overheard the neurologists talking outside his door. I was in his room at the time and heard them say, "Well, one thing is for certain . . . the paralysis is going to be permanent. . . ." At that moment this vital, wounded man looked away, his face contorted in pain. I moved forward to try to comfort him and he warded me off with his arm raised, shielding his face just like Pierre in this sculpture. I will never forget his self-contained dignity.

J. K. Jelinek

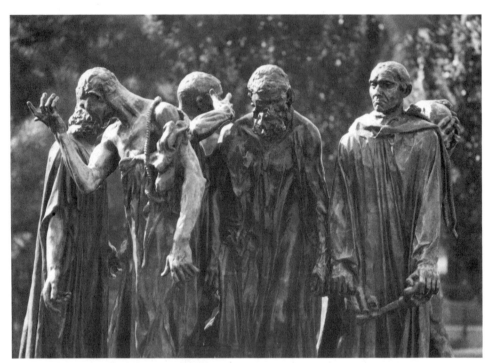

Burghers of Calais, bronze, 1884.

Rodin gave a life to each of these men in the final gesture of their life. Through his work, he has eloquently evoked compassion in the contemporary student of the human condition.

"The Burghers of Calais"

In Rodin's "Burghers of Calais," six men face the same fate of martyred death for their city. Though they express themselves dimensionally in six varied ways, Rodin has found an important truth in the unique expression of the experience each individual demonstrates.

Health professionals and nurses specifically would be enlightened to understand that these differences exist. Whether we are encountering expressions of pain, sadness, grief, resignation, anger, or frustration, we need to recognize and understand that each individual has a different experience and disposition that controls their outward expression of emotion. We then would know not to judge the emotions we encountered as contextually correct or incorrect.

Colleen Durocher

This sculpture, "The Burghers of Calais," evokes memories of my Catholic childhood and high school years spent in the parochial schools. It reminds me of the faces of Christ in many statues and sculptures seen throughout those years, especially of the time of Lent in the Catholic religious tradition. It especially evokes the depictions of Christ in the Stations of the Cross, when Christ is on His way to His death . . . carrying the cross along the road to where He is about to be executed . . . not unlike these men. I see, in each of their faces, and how different each one is, the face of Christ. Whether old and withered, young and questioning, angry, tormented, humiliated, grieving, stumbling, frightened and hopeless, they are all the faces of Christ as I remember Him portrayed in statues, pictures, and Bible passages. There is a great similarity between the Burghers and Christ, and I see those when I look at the sculpture.

When I first heard the sculpture explained, I immediately chalked it up as another story from history however many hundreds of years ago. But, as I saw the photographs, it became clear how real these men actually were. These were men with emotions and fears. I felt very sad looking at them. They evoke strong emotions. I really would like to see them in person.

Julie Vielleux

CONCLUSION

"Here is another human being, in this case a respected artist, reaching in and getting something from the viewer. This is the hallmark of art and poetry. It is not a question of the reader getting something out of the poetry. The work reaches that part of the 'readers' experience, perhaps long forgotten, that shares elements of the artist's and poet's experience. It is a unique correspondence of two strangers, and it comforts and sustains" (Hillesum, 1940). In this instance, it is the Burghers whose experience and visual representations remind us of other scenes, interactions, gestures. The Burghers are a living rosary, the chaplet, the communion between the living and the dead. As Richardson has said, "Eustache de St. Pierre has evoked a feeling of understanding and closeness for my grandfather that I never felt while he was alive."

Poetry, painting, and the arts are also attempts to find unity in the varieties of the human experience; the hidden likeness that makes our lives more vivid and unified by showing us ourselves as we are or as we might be. "It allows us to appreciate the ephemeral existence of humankind" (Anonymous, 1987).

The fleeting intangibles of human existence may seem insignificant compared to the statistical and scientific data that we are accustomed to relying upon. But a strong case can be made for focusing our attention on the realm of the intangible. All of the faculties of the soul are consciously employed in this endeavor: memory, reason, will, imagination, and the senses (sight, hearing, touch, smell, and taste).

And, finally, Rodin's masterpiece demonstrates, undisputably, that emotional states are communicated by gesture, posture, gait, indeed, all of the muscles of the body. This view educates the "clinical eye" to a sensitive view of others. For, while all of the Burghers are facing execution, each is distinctly different. Each endures his own personal reaction. And nothing other than this is possible.

The Exile of Passivity:
Kurosawa, *Ikiru*

2

Sometimes I think of my death, I think of ceasing to be . . . and it is from these thoughts that *IKIRU* came.

Akira Kurosawa, 1984

CLASS DISCUSSION

Due to the length of this film, (143 minutes, feature length), the viewing is conducted in two separate class sessions. There is a natural break in the film which occurs just as Mr. Watanabe's funeral wake begins. The first section is shown and then followed by discussion of characters, events, and film themes to this point. In the next class session, the second section is shown and is discussed in relation to the first, taking into account further events, character action, and development of theme. For the purposes of this text, these two class discussion periods will flow together so as to provide additional continuity for the reader.

Portions of the précis appeared in *Möbius* and a key note address in "Humanism, Healing and Healthcare" in Lihue, Hawaii, June 1989.

IKIRU

Akira Kurosawa. Toho/Kurosawa Productions, Japan, 1952. Japanese language with English subtitles, easily understood. May be purchased on VHS or Beta Video tape from Cinemathique Collection, Los Angeles, California, or rented as an 18mm film on two reels from Films, Inc., New York, New York.

Cast of Characters

Kanji Watanabe, Chief, Citizen's Bureau
Mitsuo, his son
Kazue, Mitsuo's wife
Kiichi, Kanji's elder brother
Tatsu, Kiichi's wife
The Maid
Ono, sub-section chief
Saito, subordinate clerk
Sakai, assistant
Kakai, assistant
Ohara, assistant
Deputy Mayor
City Councillor
Doctor
Nurse, Miss Aihara
Patient in clinic
Writer in pub
Hostess
Newspaper man
Gang Boss
Gang Member
Policeman
Housewives of Kuroe-cho
(Kurosawa, 1968)

(Continued on page 30.)

STUDENT RESPONSES

Class sessions begin with the question: Now that you have viewed this film, what did you see? What did you hear? What is your understanding of this opening scene? This excerpt from a longer discussion is presented for your review. Note the depth and variety of the responses as they unfold.

S.N.   "I was startled to see the opening scene, the X-ray negative plate showing Watanabe's cancer . . . and the narrator sounding so impersonal, calling Watanabe 'our hero,' saying he doesn't know yet that he has cancer. I immediately felt sorry for him."

S.N.   "I don't understand why his doctors could not tell him the truth. Why did he have to learn his fate from a total stranger, another patient?"

S.N.   "This stranger was a bit brutal, don't you think? Think about what he said to someone he didn't even know. And Watanabe was obviously distressed."

S.N.   "What did he say that was that bad?"

S.N.   "Well, he asks Watanabe if he has stomach trouble and tells him that he, himself, has some chronic stomach trouble. Then he launches into a description of another patient's symptoms saying, 'Now that fellow over there. They say it's ulcers but I think it's cancer. And having cancer is the same as having a death sentence. But the doctors here always tell you it's ulcers, that an operation's unnecessary. They tell you to go on and eat anything—and when you hear that, you know you've got a year left, at the most. Your stomach always feels heavy, and it hurts; you belch a lot and you're constipated or else you have diarrhoea, and in either case your stool is always black'" (Kurosawa, 1968. p. 23).

S.N.   "That scene bothered me too. I noticed that Watanabe becomes more and more uncomfortable as the man talks on, but this guy just keeps going, out of his own anxiety, I guess. He even adds, '. . . you won't be able to eat meat or anything you really like, then you'll vomit up something you ate a week ago; and when that you happens, you have about three

IKIRU (To Live) is the story of a Japanese bureaucrat, Kanji Watanabe, who learns he is going to die. This stark knowledge painfully awakens him to the fact that he has not been truly living for the last thirty years. Dulled from a monotonous petty official's life, Watanabe has drifted through life since his wife's untimely death years before. His days are endlessly filled with paper work—stamping documents with his official seal. At the Citizens Bureau he is surrounded by junior clerks who shuffle paper all day in much the same way.

When mothers of the Kuroe-cho District petition for the clearance of the swamp-infested lot in front of their homes, Watanabe is the first of many bureau chiefs in the town hall who passively send them away, passing them on to the next department. They are unwilling or unable to act.

But the shock of his impending death changes Watanabe's view of things. Visiting a medical clinic for diagnostic tests to discover the reason for his stomach troubles, he meets another patient in the waiting area. It is from him that Watanabe learns of the seriousness of his condition. This stranger discloses the symptoms of advanced stomach cancer and Watanabe recognizes them as his own. He also learns that he has just six months to live. So when he then talks with the doctor and does not hear the truth of his fate, he does not believe the advice given him. He believes the stranger's prognosis and it is shattering. However, it also serves to awaken him to life and those around him for the first time since his son was a teenager. And the results of this new awareness are not always pleasant. The knowledge that he has been a "mummy" all these years is exquisitely painful and this pain increases as he seeks comfort from his family members only to be given the most superficial of responses. Even his brother turns him away suspecting that he wants to borrow money. His son and daughter-in-law, highly suspicious of his changed behavior, think that he has a mistress. This

(*Continued on page 32.*)

months left to live' (Kurosawa, 1968, p. 23, 24). Can you imagine another patient deliberately pressing on like that knowing that the person they are telling this tale of woe to is troubled by the very same thing?"

S.N.   "I think that people sharing the horrible details of their own ailments, or their anxiety about others, is very common. Obviously, this stranger was filled with anxiety about his own fate, and he knew how ill the man he was describing had become. His fear is that this will happen to him as well. His concern is understandable, it's for himself. He doesn't grasp the fact that he is unnerving Watanabe."

S.N.   "I think that people have an inclination to share difficult physical symptoms and other occurrences with anyone who will listen. It almost seems that they gravitate to people who have the same thing, as though this person would want to know. Take, for example, what we heard in maternity the other day. A young mother-to-be was sitting in the OB-GYN Waiting Room next to another woman who had several children. And this woman was telling the young woman about her difficult labors in great detail, ignoring completely the fright she was instilling. And the young woman could not ward off the conversation."

S.N.   "Only too true, and the young woman, then, throughout all of her pregnancy has this difficult labor on her mind. And she fears this will happen to her. And I'll bet that she is not the only mother that described her difficult labor to the new mother. Probably many of her own female friends did, too."

S.N.   "While we are talking about family members, I want to voice my dismay over Watanabe's entire family; son, daughter-in-law and brother. The only one I liked at all was his sister-in-law."

S.N.   "Their behavior makes me lose faith in the notion of family. It makes me wonder just exactly what family means. Frankly, the son, Mitsuo, and his wife, Kazue, were unspeakable, shallow and self-serving. They said cruel things to him, without a care. Three times during the film Watanabe tried to tell them that he was ill, and each time they turned away from him. The image of Mr. Watanabe that first night when he came home from the clinic knowing the awful truth haunts

worries them as they have other plans for his pension fund. He realizes that he cannot find the answer he seeks with his family and turns away from them as well. He meets a writer in a local bar, a virtual stranger, who senses some great misfortune behind Watanabe's responses to him. When Watanabe discloses that he has just a few months to live and has contemplated suicide, the writer becomes intensely sympathetic to him. When he learns that Watanabe feels he cannot take this solution because he cannot figure out why he has been living all these years, the writer thinks him heroic. Watanabe wants to taste life and the writer offers to be his Mephistopheles for the evening without exacting a price.

And so, they carouse and dance the night away and even watch a strip tease dancer. Though it is apparent that this is the first time Watanabe has experienced these things and that for the moment they are distracting, ultimately they are not the antidote. This attempt at fun and forgetfulness does not work, it does not give meaning to his life.

Meanwhile, Watanabe has ceased going to work for the first time in his life. He has not even called in to say why he is not there. His commendation for 25 years of exemplary service no longer has meaning to him. And though his colleagues notice his absence and remark that, in fact, he has been unable to eat and has been seen taking medicine, they do not call or look for him. Instead they begin jousting for his position should something happen to him. It is many days before an inquiry occurs as to his whereabouts.

However, Watanabe meets Ms. Odagiri, a young clerk from the office, on the street near his home. She is looking for him to sign work release papers with his official stamp. She has found another job in a toy factory. She tells him she could no longer work at the Citizen's Bureau because of the boring routine. In his loneliness he looks to her for some companionship. The two spend the day together drinking tea, having dinner, seeing a movie. We see Watanabe smile for

(*Continued on page 34.*)

me. He is huddled alone in the dark with this awful truth, and he hears them discussing him in a very callous manner."

S.N.   "Yes, they want to build a more modern house and they need his retirement pay. They know all of the details of his savings, pension, and retirement pay. In fact, they are living in his home. He has a small room downstairs and they have the entire upper floor. Kazue wonders if her father-in-law will agree to this use of his retirement pay. Mitsuo replies, 'Well, he'll just have to live by himself if he doesn't. That will probably be the most effective way. After all, he can't take his money with him' (Kurosawa, 1968, p. 26). And the wife laughs at this!"

S.N.   "When they realize he is in the room it is too late. Watanabe is unable to speak, he is so upset, he flees the room. But rather than being ashamed at their brashness, they hold the father responsible because he was in their rooms and overheard them. And they think that despite this awful fact, he should have told them exactly why he was there and not downstairs in his room."

S.N.   "It makes you hope that this couple never has any children!"

S.N.   "Well, neither the husband nor the wife can think beyond their own comfort, they cannot reach out to this man whom they rely upon. It makes me wonder what their day-to-day life was before this incident. Were they living in just this way? Did they always ignore the father? Are they totally preoccupied with themselves?"

S.N.   "Right, didn't the father ever ask anything of them? I mean, didn't they ever talk?"

S.N.   "It's possible that they lived, say, task-oriented lives that were as monotonous and dull as Watanabe's. Don't forget the opening scenes of the film. Watanabe is sitting amongst piles and piles of files, stamping documents. All of his assistants sit at a long row of desks doing the very same thing. He hasn't missed a day of work in 25 years!"

S.N.   "He was barely living."

S.N.   "Later in the film, we see his son at work, and he is sitting amongst a bunch of co-workers at a long row of desks, doing paper work."

S.N.   "The father, son, and daughter-in-law were already alienated from one another long before this incident. Otherwise it

the first time while talking to her. In fact, he becomes animated and solicitous of her.

He continues to seek her out but she becomes nervous that he might be in love with her and he is too old. She does not grasp his desperate need for companionship and becomes frightened of his intenseness. In their last meeting there is a confrontation as he tells her he is dying. She is repelled by this news and cannot understand what she can do. But Watanabe presses and tells her that facing death alone is like the time when he was a young child and nearly drowned and his parents were very far away. He realizes in one sense that nothing can save him and yet, in another sense, he can be saved if he can find a reason for having lived—if he could live one day fully as she does. In her youth she does not know what to tell him, but to her credit she stays with him even though she now is quite frightened. She blurts out that she just goes to work and makes toy rabbits. This makes her feel as though she is friends with all of the children of Japan.

These words provide the clue that gives him the idea of how "to live," what will give meaning and purpose to his life. His thought is to find the forgotten petition of the mothers of Kuroe-cho. He will force through the bureaucratic walls of obstinacy and build a park in place of the infested swamp. In this plan he is very determined, and he is a changed man when he returns to work—persistent, quietly confrontative—fighting personal discouragement and physical pain. At one point he is roughed up and intimidated by gangsters who want the area for a bar. But in his dogged persistence he is able to force the park into being. It is this commitment to others that gives meaning to his life.

never would have occurred. If they had been close and had then found him in such distress, they would have tried to find out why. And, they never would have been having that awful conversation."

S.N. "Toward the end of the film, Watanabe remarks to Kimura, his assistant, that he has not seen a sunset for 25 years. They are standing on the bridge overlooking the city. This is another indication that he has been living a monotonous, dull existence . . . maybe even a depressed one."

S.N. "It is frightening to think that a life can become so dulled that family relationships fall away and they don't even notice the changing weather. It's an awful passivity or something. Just about everyone in City Hall was afflicted with it, too."

S.N. "A case in point is the very first day that the mothers of the Kuroe-cho District come to complain about the swamp-infested land in front of their dwellings. It is infested with mosquitoes, and the children are getting ill, they cannot play out in their own front yards. The clerk that they ask for assistance tells them he cannot help, it must come under sanitation. So they try the Health Centre. Sanitation Section then sends them to Environmental Health Section. Once there they are sent to Pest Control Section, and so on until the women become very weary of this charade and angrily assert themselves, 'What do you think we are anyway? What does this sign mean? Isn't this your responsibility?'" (Kurosawa, 1968, p. 22)

S.N. "This is a very clear picture of bureaucratic passivity that leads to inaction. These people are not doing the work that the bureau was created to do!"

S.N. "They have a remarkable way of passing the buck from one department to the next."

S.N. "It reminds me of trying to straighten out financial aid up at our administration building."

S.N. "This actually reminds me of what our patients endure when they come into the medical center trying to understand what is happening to them."

S.N. "Yes, they try to get blood studies and X-rays, and other diagnostic tests. And, of course, they can't find out the results right away."

S.N.   "These scenes in the film are very much like what the poor are up against when they try to get any assistance in any institution."

S.N.   "This also happens all of the time for the elderly. They get piles and piles of bills, sometimes double bills. And they have to try to figure out what all of these insurance companies want. I saw one elderly woman's collection of bills after her husband was hospitalized. She had two shopping bags full of mail from different hospitals and insurance companies. It's awful. She would call these different financial offices or companies trying to get help. They would pass her on from one to the next, endlessly. She was very, very discouraged."

S.N.   "Partly, I'll bet because some of the companies don't honor what they say they will."

S.N.   "This is the way it is, this 'passing the buck' in most institutions. Sometimes it makes you feel kind of hopeless."

S.N.   "You have to expect institutions to be like that, that's just the way it is."

S.N.   "I don't think that is true, but it takes someone out of the ordinary to cut through that nonsense."

S.N.   "That means someone who has some sympathy for the person standing in front of them and that person needs to be consciously aware of others."

S.N.   "The doctors and the nurse fall into this same category because they basically lie to Watanabe the day of his diagnostic tests. I am beginning to see that they, in part, are just being self-protective."

S.N.   "But remember in the Moyer's film *Medicine East and West*, Japanese doctors did not tell patients when they had cancer because they were afraid that they would lose hope."

S.N.   "But that's ridiculous! Watanabe already knew! He was in pain, he couldn't eat! He even said to them 'Be honest with me. Tell me the truth. Tell me it's cancer.' (Kurosawa, 1968, p. 24). Instead, the doctor replies, 'Not at all. It's just a light case of ulcers, as I said' (Kurosawa, 1968, p. 24). Watanabe wants to know, 'Is an operation impossible?' (Kurosawa, 1968, p. 24). He is told it is unnecessary, that medicine will fix him up and he can eat anything he likes as long as it's digestible."

S.N.   "You're right, and the fact that the doctor says exactly what the patient in the waiting room has already told him means that Watanabe knew he was going to die soon. You could see the terror in his face."

S.N.   "But the doctors didn't know that the patient in the waiting room told Watanabe anything."

S.N.   "Still, I think that the doctors and the nurses betrayed him. After all, they blatantly lied to him, either by commission or omission. Really, what if he believed them? What if he hadn't run into that stranger?"

S.N.   "It's true. His life is not theirs, his body is not theirs. His fate is not theirs to hide. He deserves, no, it is more than he deserves, he has the right to know what someone has learned about his body, or his mind, for that matter."

S.N.   "Besides, his life is already hopeless; he needs hope—he needs to find a reason to live!"

S.N.   "I agree with what you said about people having the right to know what others find out about them, including psychological testing. No matter how ill they are."

S.N.   "Actually, you can tell that the doctors and the nurse do not believe in hope. Otherwise they would know that telling someone that they have less than six months to live might mean something different to that person. And, I think, they are acting according to their own inability to face death and their own state of hopelessness."

S.N.   "I agree. When the chief doctor asks the nurse, Miss Aihaira, what she would do if she had only half a year to live, she answers without hesitation, 'Well, there's some poison there on the shelf'" (Kurosawa, 1968, p. 24).

S.N.   "Wow! I caught that, too. It was scary to think that a nurse might think that about herself, or her patients."

S.N.   "What do you mean? After all, maybe she just didn't want to suffer."

S.N.   "Well, I think that it is upsetting to think that if you have a fatal illness you might just as well kill yourself."

S.N.   "Some people who are in health care today might think along those same lines. You know, if you're going to be in terrible pain and use up all kinds of resources, and you only have a few months to live . . . well, some people really do think along those lines."

S.N.   "I think that there are enough ways to deal with severe pain so that a person shouldn't have to think that way or endure such a thing."

S.N.   "The thing that bothers me about this is that people are left with awful pain; not everyone seems to know what to do."

S.N.   "I don't believe it is up to us to decide such things! And besides, people do lots of things that are important to them, and to others, when they find out that they don't have much longer to live."

S.N.   "That is certainly true of the man in this film. He doesn't want to die yet, even though he is in a lot of pain. And you can tell he is really scared."

S.N.   "But he never seems to forget it for a moment, that he doesn't have much time left."

S.N.   "He doesn't have trouble facing the truth."

S.N.   "It's not so much that he doesn't have trouble but more that he seeks it out anyway."

S.N.   "Here's what I think. I think that the actual emotion that the 'truth teller' has when they tell someone something awful may be an indicator of some kind."

S.N.   "How so?"

S.N.   "Just that maybe how they felt when they are 'telling' should indicate to them whether they should be 'telling.' Look, the man in this film felt better after he told Watanabe 'the truth.' And the mother in the OB-GYN Waiting Room felt better after she told about her difficult labors."

S.N.   "I think that they did so because they were scared or maybe, in the mother's case, because she just needed to talk about it even though it had happened quite awhile ago."

S.N.   "Maybe that's why there was some excitement in their voices when they 'told the truth'."

S.N.   "So, how are they any different from the doctors and the nurse in this story? Maybe they were kinder."

S.N.   "No. I think that it wasn't so much that they didn't want to destroy Watanabe's hope, they were afraid to tell."

S.N.   "And, they were just as much institutional bureaucrats as doctors, like Watanabe himself. They had lost a sense of dealing with human beings."

S.N.   "Well, this is the way it happens in Japan, not in the States. American health care professionals are educated to be truthful in these situations."

S.N.   "I don't agree. I've seen the doctors come in on rounds and really fudge when the patients ask them direct questions. They try very hard to avoid serious discussions then. Some promise to come back later and they do. But some don't."

S.N.   "It's the same with the relatives at times. They are desperate for answers, they're so scared. And they don't always get those answers."

S.N.   "You know, when Watanabe leaves the hospital that day, he looks like he is in shock. He walks out the front door right into moving traffic. He doesn't even hear the noise that the cars and trucks are making, he doesn't even see them."

S.N.   "That's what terrible news does, how it effects you . . . you do not hear or see the same as before."

S.N.   "It is an amazing fact to me that he gets comforted by another total stranger."

S.N.   "Personally, I think that writer in the pub was one weird fellow. He may have felt sorry for Watanabe but he was more interested in what he could learn from someone who had little time left."

S.N.   "I see Ms. Odagiri quite differently. She wasn't exactly a stranger but they did not really know one another."

S.N.   "I think that she was more conscious than most of the men in the film. She knew very early in her life that she could not tolerate the atmosphere of the Bureau, and she resigned. Why she couldn't even get them to laugh at witty jokes."

S.N.   "Do you remember, when Mr. Watanabe grabs her toy rabbit and runs out of the coffee shop, you can hear the strains of the "Happy Birthday" song in the background? In a way, it was his birthday, because it was then that he began to feel alive."

S.N.   "Alive because he was trying to help the mothers of Kuroe-cho get their park."

S.N.   "But I don't think he felt guilty for all those years he worked in the Bureau, do you? After all, he didn't commit graft or anything."

S.N.   "Yes! Of course! He does feel guilt or remorse or something like that because he was so passive. He was the Chief of the Citizen's Bureau and he did little to truly help the citizens."

S.N.   "Are you implying, then, that a person has to become fatally ill before they become morally conscious? If so, I don't agree because there are many things that can penetrate people, that arouse them to care about others, and cause them to worry about their own behavior."

S.N.   "Like what?"

S.N.   "It could be, for instance, an involvement in a profession, or something deep that they have read, or sometimes it is personal loss."

S.N.   "For Watanabe, though, it is the horrible realization that he is going to die and he wakes up to the fact that to that point his life has been meaningless."

S.N.   "There are lots of people who hear that stark message and never have any revelation like that. They never change one single thing in their lives."

S.N.   "Maybe they were already conscious."

S.N.   "Perhaps."

S.N.   "We are not in the position of judging whether or not someone's life has been morally responsible."

S.N.   "I don't think that that is what I am implying. I know I'm young but it's just that the few individuals that I have been with who were dying didn't seem to examine their lives the way Watanabe did. One had his relatives running non-stop catering to him and the other just retreated into a kind of angry despair, lashing out at absolutely everyone."

S.N.   "Well, one question we could ask ourselves is whether or not we will be like the nurse and doctors in this film. What will we do when someone as needy as Watanabe confronts us begging for help?"

S.N.   "Will we even hear the clues to this big question he asked 'Why have I been living?'"

S.N.   "We have, in a way, already asked ourselves something like that. We chose to become nurses. We can hardly be passive in the face of that."

S.N.   "Oh, that's not true. There are many different ways to be passive in the health care arena. For instance, it is easy to 'pass the buck' when someone is very upset. And we do it out of self protection, or maybe fear because we don't know what to say or do."

S.N.   "One of the phrases I have heard a lot since we have been going to our clinical sites is 'Well, we have never done this or that like that before and we can't change now.'"

S.N.   "There are some nurses out there who really would prefer, still, to be the 'old hand-maiden to the doc' rather than take responsibility for their own practice."

S.N.   "Easier said than done!"

S.N.   "It's hard to take that enormous responsibility. Everything is against you. There is never enough time, staffing is always awful. The patients are a lot sicker. And now there has been all of this restructuring going on. Really, nurses are being let go and untrained 'technicians' are being hired."

S.N.   "I was told by a registered nurse who has been working at the medical center for years, 'Just you wait, you will lose your idealism when you graduate and join the real world.' She was very angry when she said this and it was because I had insisted on remaining with a family and she had other plans for me. I tried to explain why I thought that this was important to the family but she would hear none of it."

S.N.   "Just as there are all kinds of bureaucrats, there are all kinds of nurses and there is just so much thoughtless behavior that can be excused."

S.N.   "It seems to me what we are saying is that we want to be someone who does not look for excuses for not acting."

S.N.   "Kimura, Watanabe's assistant wanted to be like him."

S.N.   "But when he was tested in the end, after the wake, when the mothers sought help at the Bureau, he couldn't act. He tried, but he couldn't in the face of all of the other workers who passively sat and watched."

S.N. "The wake spelled it all out. Everyone tries to understand what happened to Watanabe, why he died. After they debunk the Deputy Mayor's claim that he was the one who created the park in Kuroe-cho, they try to figure out where all of Watanabe's new found courage came from."

S.N. "They were told that he died of a hemorrhage due to gastric cancer. But they cannot figure out now this gave him courage."

S.N. "During the wake I found myself getting hopeful that Kimura would follow in Watanabe's footsteps. He seemed to understand the needs of the people. He felt a kinship with Watanabe. I felt sad, too, that he crumbled."

S.N. "In light of our discussion about what it takes to become a person of conscience, I think that we should look at the fact that none of these men have confronted their own responsibility towards Watanabe. They feel no real guilt for ignoring his obvious pain, or his long absence from work. They have no trouble angling for his job when he dies. I think they hoped he wouldn't return."

S.N. "I think they felt a momentary pang of guilt, but it was when they were drunk on sake."

S.N. "I must say, I object to the moral overtones of this conversation. We are here to learn about nursing not to get a catechism lesson. Listen to the way you all are talking! This is depressing. We can't keep track of all of these things for our patients."

S.N. "I think that it is worthwhile to try to understand the inner forces that motivate people. For instance, look at the characters in this film. I don't think that we should be quick to judge, or judge at all. But, the way that the co-workers and relatives reacted to Mr. Watanabe's illness does tell you something about them. And I can't help but think that their ability to face things out would affect their own health one day. I should add, inability, since most of these people turned away from him."

S.N. "Right! The only one who did not was Ms. Odigiri. I think she had integrity. She was always very candid with him even when he frightened her. She seemed to have a respect for herself that the others did not have."

S.N.   "I think that the sister-in-law had some dignity, too. She wanted to help Watanabe but her husband was very mocking of her, and of his own brother."

S.N.   "The writer could face the truth, he proved that. It's just that his solution to drink and have a good time watching the stripper didn't work."

S.N.   "It's simply true, everyone would react differently to the news that Watanabe got, and not all would be as brave as he was."

S.N.   "I know, remember at the end of the film, after the wake, Mitsuo, his son, finds a box with his father's bank book, the plaque honoring his 25 years of meritorious service to the Citizen's Bureau, a clock and the toy rabbit. Now, to me, that is a very telling legacy, very symbolic. But his son doesn't understand at all. Not even after he learns that his father forced the park into being against great odds."

S.N.   "Also, he must have suspected that his father did know about the stomach cancer."

S.N.   "But his reaction is one of anger and disappointment with his father."

S.N.   "He will never see how he affects others, only how they affect him. Well, maybe never is too strong a word, but I think there is a very slim chance that he will ever feel as fulfilled as his father did the night that he died in the park."

CONCLUSION

Kurosawa uses many techniques to awaken us to Watanabe's plight; fascinating details, flashbacks, music, and narrative. In fact, throughout the film are strains of American music and the big band sound, showing the effects of American culture on Japan in the early fifties. Kurosawa uses every available means to force us to feel what Watanabe feels in order to alert us to the dangers of passivity in our personal lives. He is very clear about the sacrifices that become necessary when one begins to fight to remain conscious—to live fully oneself and compassionately on behalf of others. He is telling us that it is possible to break out of meaningless routine. This is preventive medicine, beginning with compassion for oneself.

Following are two student stories written in response to the theme in the film which led the students to conclude that the doctors and the nurse in the story were "just institutional bureaucrats, like Watanabe, himself. They had lost the sense of dealing with human beings."

Not Questioning
by Arthur Sullivan

She was lying on the treatment table trying desperately to move her head from side to side. High pitched cries pierced the atmosphere. She was eight months old. But they were ineffective in gaining an end to the treatment. I was trying to calm her with a soothing voice, hoping she might hear it in her semisedated state. I held her head tightly, the length of my hands were large enough to encircle the entire circumference of her tiny head, while the surgeon probed the open wound in her neck.

Generously lending the clean white roll of tape that I kept looped through by stethoscope ear pieces, I had helped others to tape the child to the table, two strips across the legs, and one across her small chest. I silently, but sarcastically, laughed at the situation, and at the nurses trying to practice aseptic technique. The surgeon, lost in his own world, had picked up the sterile gloves with both of his hands, contaminating almost all of the sterile equipment. He did not want to take the time to open the proper incision and drainage kit. His actions did not phase me. Since starting nursing school two years before, I had frequently seen poor technique by physicians; they were always rushed and on a mission, forgetting to take into account the intricacies of patients' needs.

I stood by, silent, guilty, realizing that I had become apathetic towards advocating for the patient, as had the other two nurses in the room. I rationalized my silence by the fact that I was a student nurse in my junior year, powerless to bring about change in a system whose practices were decades old and ingrained in stone. Through my recent clinical experiences I had become jaded, no longer naive or idealistic. To tell this seasoned physician how to practice sterile technique would be to rock the health care boat that theoretically sailed so calmly along, and to become a trouble maker and an enemy in the eyes of the staff. An instigator of change is seen as a threat, forcing all to consciously examine their own behavior, possibly deducing that they might need to work harder to preserve human dignity and care.

I was physically at the table, but withdrawn at the same time, swimming in an ocean of discombobulated thoughts and emotions. I tried to reach deep inside for some inkling of personal sorrow or sympathy for the situation, for the little girl, but to no avail. I wanted to feel the way I did in the beginning of my clinical training. During that period, there was more than one time that I wept uncontrollably at others' suffering. And I always felt a deep personal bond with the patients. I was determined to be part of a medical and nursing staff that wanted to offer themselves completely to the care and healing of ill individuals. I made a vow to advocate for the patient, to stand up, to initiate change in the system, even if this meant being a martyr of sorts. How could I have changed so drastically in such a short time, transformed from a truly compassionate, idealistic nurse, into an individual that seemed to have lost the ability to care?

My mind drifted back to the treatment room. I glanced at the strips of taut white tape, and then at the dark black hair on my rough broad tensed hands, the veins raised from the firm grip on the baby's tiny pale face. I watched as a shiny steel probe darted in and out of the incision, and then a scalpel; any tool available was considered adequate. Small amounts of stringy yellow necrotic tissue was pulled from the large opening, and the surgeon seemed aggravated as he mumbled "I want pus." My mind continued to pay tribute to my past. Questions and ideas oozed forth, struggling to address the possible ramification of my personal changes as a student nurse and as a human being. In awe, without forewarning, I had arrived at this present state and was now fearstruck with the thought of the unpredictability of my future.

The Silent Patient
by Christine Molloy

As the student nurse entered the Tauma Intensive Unit she felt excited. All semester she had been looking forward to her two-day rotation here. Now she was almost overwhelmed with anticipation combined with fear. These feelings lingered as she entered her patient's room. This was going to be very different from any of her other medical-surgical experiences.

The initial shock of seeing the patient for the first time hit her pretty hard. He was a big man and he was rotating back and forth on a Roto-rest Kinetic Bed. He seemed almost lost among all of the wires and machines that surrounded. The student recognized the ventilator, EKG machine, and the IV pole. But the IV pole had four or five lines coming from it with all kinds of medications in the collection of bottles. The amount of technology in that one room stunned her. Then another stark reality hit her; this wasn't a patient who was going to sit up and talk to her. This was someone in a coma, supported by machines, hovering between life and death.

"You might as well come over and listen to the report," the registered nurse called out to her, bringing her back to the reality of the room.

"This is a fifty-one year old police officer involved in a hit-and-run accident late last night," began the nurse. While listening to the report, the student nurse learned that there was a real story attached to Phil.

"He has a complete fracture in his right leg where the tibia and fibula connect, severe lacerations in the right parietal lobe with an excessive amount of subarachnoid hemorrhaging. There is also a question of fractured vertebrae. They have to take some more X-Rays today," she added.

As the night nurse finished the physical report of this patient, she began to speak about the social aspects of his life. Apparently, according to the nurse, Phil had ended a love affair with another woman several months previously. However, when he was admitted to the hospital, she showed up and demanded to see him saying that they were still together. The wife was there at the time and was absolutely devastated. Compounding this drama was the man's mother who somehow blamed the situation on the wife because Phil was working overtime "to support her materialism."

This private information was being transmitted over the comatose police officer, lying motionless, unable to communicate yet possibly able to comprehend everything going on around him, or so the student imagined.

After giving the report the night nurse prepared to leave and the day nurse began her assessment.

"What a bastard," she said as she looked at the picture the wife had put up in the room of their family.

"What did you say?" the student asked incredulously.

"He's a bastard. His wife gives him another chance and look what he does to her, he screws her over. She's been at the hospital all night praying for him and he doesn't deserve it. He doesn't deserve her either."

Everyone seemed to treat the man mechanically, the student thought. They didn't speak to him, just attended to his physiological needs and continued to assess his status.

His wife tearfully begged him to try to move, "Please honey, just move your hand, something . . . anything." The student imagined his thoughts were racing as he concentrated all of his efforts on moving his finger. She was sure that he was trying to communicate. Perhaps he wanted to tell his wife how sorry he was. And maybe he wanted to tell those nurses that they had no right to judge him. And then, he did it, he made his little finger move back and forth. "Oh my God, I knew it!" the wife exclaimed, she had felt the finger twitch.

When the nurse came back, she told her that she had felt her husband move his little finger. She wanted to know if this meant that he was regaining consciousness. "Probably not," the nurse replied coolly. "He has minimal brain activity right now and it was probably an after-effect of stopping the Norucuron infusions."

Again the student imagined the man thinking, "How frustrating this is!"

The student nurse had been following the registered nurse as she tended to the patients. She assisted whenever she could. But she was bothered by what she had seen and heard. She felt a distance between her and the nurses. She could not accept what they had said about this man. She didn't like what he had done, but he was suffering. Why couldn't they value that?

During her coffee break, the student returned to the man's room. Embarrassed but steadfast, she felt that she had to speak to this man. Yet, she felt uncomfortable treating a comatose man as though he were awake. But she did talk to him. And as she talked, she became more comfortable. A strange feeling overcame her, she was sure that he could hear her. Then she realized that throughout the morning, she had never touched him humanly. Everytime she had touched him she had had gloves on. Removing them she gently took his hand and was surprised at the warmth she felt.

"Yes, I'm alive, I'm fighting," he seemed to say.

The warmth of his hand reassured her somehow. Maybe it was her imagination. Maybe she was just a naive student nurse with too much hope. But she knew that he felt her presence somehow. She couldn't explain it to anybody. She didn't even understand it and she didn't expect anyone else to either. She could only describe it as a feeling, a feeling that some sort of communication had taken place and that she had made a difference in his life, as he had in hers.

3

The Exile of
Abandonment:
Sophocles, *Philoktetes*

The aim of tragedy is to express and call forth a collective sympathy with ideal sorrow, and thus, while relieving and enlarging the heart, and refining and elevating its emotions, to infix and deepen the truths of the human experience.

Lewis Campbell, 1874

STUDENT ARGUMENTS

Prior to class, students closely read and annotated the play. There are natural breaking points within the play which lend themselves to extended discussion. When the class meets, students read the play aloud, arguing for or against a character's behavior. They try to understand the perspective of the characters and the reasons for their actions. Students are asked to consider the persons in the drama as

Portions of the précis appeared in the *Journal of Professional Nursing* and a research presentation at the Sigma Theta Tau International Research Congress in Edinburgh, Scotland, July 1987.

PHILOKTETES

Sophocles. (408 b.c.) Translated by Gregory McNamee (1986) Washington: Copper Canyon Press.

The Persons

Odysseus, general of the Achaean Troops

Neoptolemus, teenaged son of the recently slain Achilles

Chorus of Mariners

Philoktetes, recruited by Achaean generals to serve in war against Troy, bequeathed Heracles' magical bow

Messenger, disguised as Merchantman, actually a spy

Heracles, a demi god, appearing from the sky

Scene, a desert shore of the Island of Lemnos, uninhabited

(During the discussion students are encouraged to quote directly from the drama in order to emphasize points they wish to analyze. Note the depth and variety of the responses as they unfold.)

PHILOKTETES (The Philoctetean myth first appeared in the Little Iliad) is a play about an outcast who was abandoned on an un-inhabited island for 10 years until his talent as a warrior and his unique possession of Hercules' bow and arrow were needed to turn the tide of the Trojan War. Bitten by a viper 10 years before while leading his soldiers to a shrine, Philoktetes developed a wound that would not heal and by which he was crippled. His incessant cries of agony and complaint and the malodorous wound were unbearable to his comrades in the Greek Army. Encouraged by Odysseus, they deserted him on the Isle of Lemnos. There, living in a cave, he endured

(Continued on page 52.)

archetypal guides for understanding the implications for truth telling. For the purposes of this text, each character's behavior, as it occurs throughout the drama, will be discussed in kind.

S.N.   "Some say that Odysseus is a thoughtless or conniving man. But lots of the things that he says and does can be taken two ways. For instance, in the opening scene he tries to explain why he deserted Philoktetes on Lemnos:

> *I had to cast him away here:*
> *our masters, the kings, commanded me to,*
> *for disease had conquered him, and his foot*
> *was eaten away by festering sores.*
> *We had no recourse. At our holy feasts,*
> *we could not reach for meat and wine.*
> *He would not let us sleep;*
> *he howled all night, wilder than a wolf.*
> *He blanketed our camp with evil cries,*
> *moaning and screaming.*

(McNamee, p. 9)

S.N.   "Right. He was commanded to do it back then because his king made him do it. Apparently, they could not celebrate holy feasts properly."

S.N.   "But, he gives the real clues as to why he did it . . . he can't stand Philoktetes' complaining, he can't stand to hear his moaning and crying."

S.N.   "Well, before he left him there on a deserted island, he did find him just the right place—a cave with two openings, exposed to the sun:

> *for warmth in the cold months,*
> *admitting cool breezes in summer's heat;*
> *to the left, nearby it, a sweet-running spring.*

(McNamee, p. 10)

loneliness, extremes of weather, hunger, and unremitting pain. His torment was further intensified by sailors to the Isle who refused him passage home.

Odysseus and Neoptolemus, Achilles' young son, traveled to Lemnos to trick Philoktetes into coming back to Greece with the Herculean bow and arrow. A captured oracle, Helanos has warned them that they will be unable to win the war without the magical bow (McNamee, 1986). They feel justified in the devious mission, though Neoptolemus argues that trickery is dishonorable. Odysseus cunningly reasons with the young man using the ploy that 'lying for gain is not shameful in the affairs of state—when it is for the greater good' (Campbell, 1847). In order to win the Trojan War, they must have Philoktetes and the famed bow and arrow.

Once Neoptolemus has gained the faith of Philoktetes, the two make preparations to leave Lemnos. Suddenly Philoktetes is overwhelmed with a paroxysm of pain; his festering wound has erupted anew and the pain is so agonizing that he begs Neoptolemus to shear off his foot. Neoptolemus is filled with genuine concern for the suffering man, but is frightened and does not know what to do. Philoktetes beseeches him, "Do not, in fear, forsake me." Neoptolemus does stay to console him; in the process of this shared suffering he becomes ashamed of his duplicity. He realizes that he must honor this forsaken man's faith in him. He confesses the deceitful plot to Philoktetes, who is enjoying a long awaited reprieve from his lonely miseries. This newest betrayal heaped upon so many others over the past 10 years is too great for him to bear. The consoling justice that he craved, and now thought was his, has vanished. In his torment he threatens to kill Odysseus and then himself. It is only when Neoptolemus defies Odysseus in order to honor his word to the desperate man that confidence is restored. (Young-Mason, 1988, p. 299)

S.N.   "What he remembers about what he did is very different from what actually happened because Philoktetes describes the place a lot differently and he lived there.

> *I have had to make my own life,*
> *to be my own servant in this tiny cave.*
> *I seek out birds to fill by stomach,*
> *and shoot them down.*
> *After I let loose a tautly drawn bolt,*
> *I drag myself along on this stinking foot.*
> *When I had to drink the water that pours from this spring,*
> *in icy winter, I had to break up wood,*
> *crippled as I am,*
> *and melt the ice alone.*
> *I dragged myself around and did it.*
> *And if the fire went out, I had to sit,*
> *and grind stone against stone*
> *until a spark sprang up to save my life.*
> *This roof, if I have fire, at least gives me a home,*
> *gives me all I need to stay alive*
> *except release from my anguish.*

(McNamee, p. 22, 23)

S.N.   "Anyway, it is very wrong to desert someone who is in such a wounded state."

S.N.   "Odysseus acts as though if you just give someone who has been hurt, or has some disease a decent place to live you aren't neglecting them."

S.N.   "Also, he decides what is decent and since he doesn't really care about what happens to him, he isn't concerned about the fact that the place might be too cold or that the food would be hard to get. He just doesn't care."

S.N.   "Well, the story gets worse. He has Neoptolemus looking for him now that he is needed to help win the war with the magic bow. They can't find him but they do find the cave and they see the rags that he used for bandages drying in the sun."

S.N. "I think that Odysseus does know how bad off Philoktetes is because of what he says when they don't find him in the cave:

> *He can't be far off.*
> *Weakened as he is by long years of disease,*
> *he can't stray far from home.*

(McNamee, p. 11)

S.N. "He is even sarcastic, he adds:

> *He is probably out scratching up a meal*
> *or an herb he knows will relieve his pain.*

(McNamee, p. 11)

S.N. "This is every bit the way it is today. Last week a young couple on welfare was sent home with their newborn baby within 24 hours of its birth. Nobody checked to see what the living circumstances were in their apartment. They were just glad that they had a place to go to. We would never have known if I had not been sent out on a home visit. I had stayed with this young woman throughout her labor and delivery, so I got to go on the home visit. Well, I was blown away. First of all, they lived in a very rough neighborhood in a dilapidated house with lots of other families. The place was five stories high. But, when I was actually let into the apartment I really had a shock. They had absolutely nothing! Not even a bed, or a crib, or table, chairs, nothing. There was no refrigerator, not even hot running water. I thought that I was going there to help with the baby's first bath and that sort of thing. But that was the least of what they needed. Really, they needed everything. And when I talked with the head nurse about this she said, 'That's the way it is—that's the real world.'"

S.N. "But they weren't sick or wounded or anything like that."

S.N. "No, they weren't sick—yet. They were just poor."

S.N. "You can get cast out by society if you are really sick, or really poor, either one."

S.N. "How so?"

S.N. "It makes a difference which disease you have."

S.N.   "What are you getting at?"

S.N.   "If you have a disease that you can be blamed for you are in for it."

S.N.   "Such as?"

S.N.   "Number one on that list is AIDS. Now I am not saying that everyone turns away from individuals who have AIDS. It makes a difference whether or not the person got it directly from another person, you know, by sexual transmission or drug use, or if they got it through a blood transfusion."

S.N.   "And then there is lung cancer in a smoker, or cirrhosis of the liver in an alcoholic. These people are held accountable for their own health problems."

S.N.   "I hate to admit it but I don't see why these people should get the same attention as those who have taken care of themselves all of their lives."

S.N.   "I would like to add that people with severe mental illness are in the same category as those who have AIDS or cancer or cirrhosis."

S.N.   "The poor, the disenfranchised don't have means to care for themselves."

S.N.   "I am not saying that everyone in health care treats people this way, necessarily, but I do say that lots of health care professionals get angry at this sort of patient. People who carry on like Philoktetes did are a real bother."

S.N.   "I have seen that all right. There was a young woman at the medical center who had AIDS, and she was in the end stages of the illness. She had open sores that really hurt and she had to nearly beg nurses to come into her room just to put vaseline on her lips. She was too weak to do it herself."

S.N.   "I don't see the nurses behaving as badly as Odysseus here. After all, they could have been extremely busy, they might not have heard her."

S.N.   "But *I* heard her cries and I was at the other end of the hall!"

S.N.   "I don't think that nurses think like Odysseus, they don't purposefully ignore wounded people or set them aside or send them away. You are talking about desertion here, that's what Odysseus did, he deserted Philoktetes."

S.N.   "Not only that, he gets word that he is never going to win this Trojan War, and it has been going on for 10 years, unless he finds Philoktetes. And he only wants him now because he has the famous 'magic bow.'"

S.N. "His actions are in keeping with his character. All along he shades the truth. When he deserted him 10 years before, he and the whole army stopped at the island of Lemnos. He waited until Philoktetes fell asleep and then they all snuck off. They left him there all alone."

S.N. "And now he needs him back again for the bow, so he hatches a little plan of deception that is especially bad."

S.N. "Philoktetes never would have gone with him after what he did."

S.N. "Why is it so much worse than other things that he has done?"

S.N. "Because he gets his dead friend's son to be an accomplice. The son is just a teenager."

S.N. "At first he was easily taken in, but he is never for the plot that Odysseus hatches."

S.N. "Odysseus is very persuasive and he tries to convince Neoptolemus that, and this is a great phrase, 'the end justifies the means'" (McNamee, p. 13).

S.N. "He admits that if Philoktetes saw him he would try to kill him. But he knows Philoktetes will befriend the son of his comrade. He tells him that the taking of Troy depends on his ability to lie cleverly. So, Neoptolemus must convince Philoktetes that he hates him (Odysseus).

> *Say whatever you want to*
> *against me, Say the worst that comes to mind.*
> *None of it will insult me. If you do not match this task,*
> *you will cast endless sorrow and suffering on the Greeks.*
>
> (McNamee, p. 12)

S.N. "He even appeals to Neoptolemus' honor saying:

> *I know son, that by nature you are unsuited*
> *to tell such lies and work such evil.*
> *But the prize of victory is a sweet thing to have.*
>
> (McNamee, p. 12)

S.N.   "This action has parallels to today. We had a patient in the unit who was homeless. He had awful sores all over his body and he had burned both of his feet really badly. They were all infected. He was in a lot of pain and screamed all of the time, called the nurses and doctors names I wouldn't repeat. He even threw a tray of food at the wall in his room. Nobody seemed to be able to deal with him. Everybody was trying to hatch some plot to get him to leave the hospital, to go somewhere else to get treated."

S.N.   "I know who that is, he really needed to be in the hospital, he was very sick."

S.N.   "What bothered me was they were giving him all kinds of reasons to leave and some of them were threatening, like 'We simply have to have peace and quiet for the other patients to get well,' or, 'If you don't appreciate how we are trying to help you, you should go somewhere else.'"

S.N.   "One group got onto the fact that he caused his own problems because he drank. They said that he fell asleep one night when he was drunk and that's how his feet got burned. Therefore he was to blame and should behave . . . he was causing the whole staff a lot of unnecessary work and grief."

S.N.   "I've heard that reasoning about difficult patients before. Part of me feels sorry for the person no matter what happened and part of me has a lot of sympathy for the nurses and doctors."

S.N.   "Just the same, if you put yourself in this guy's place it must be awfully scarey, he can't behave and he can't get better."

S.N.   "You're right about that because the staff senior resident discharged him against his will, in a way, and he was too embarrassed to fight them."

S.N.   "Who would want to stay with the whole staff against them?"

S.N.   "Ugh! I've never heard of such a thing, a sick person being thrown out of a hospital."

S.N.   "Where have you been? It happens all of the time. Maybe not because they are bad, sometimes it's because their insurance runs out."

S.N.   "Oh, I know about that sort of thing, but I mean cases like this guy having to leave because nobody could deal with him."

S.N.   "I wonder what happens to people like that."

S.N. "I don't get the analogy between this guy and Philoktetes, after all, nobody was trying to deceive this homeless guy."

S.N. "I think it's a bigger lie than Odysseus' to Philoktetes because what happened to this guy makes the idea of getting care in a hospital a joke, a mockery."

S.N. "They did send in a social worker to try to get him to behave so that he could stay. But I don't think that she ever found out why he was so angry."

S.N. "So, don't you see? When they threatened him with having to leave and then executed their plan, they were deserting him just like Philoktetes was deserted, and for similar reasons."

S.N. "Right, they didn't even take him somewhere, they just put him out on the street."

S.N. "Maybe they assumed he was going to the homeless shelter."

S.N. "There are other kinds of lies that seem, when they are told, to be for the best. You know, the end justifies the means kind of thing. We had a woman with lung disease who refused to try to wean herself off of the respirator even though her doctor thought she could breathe on her own. The staff had a case conference and decided to shut off the respirator without telling her. They thought they would be able to show her that she could actually do it. But she easily guessed what they were up to and she was terrified. She got to the point where she was too afraid to go to sleep because she was certain that they would shut it off then and she wouldn't be able to breathe at all."

S.N. "It seems to me that the situations that we have been talking about are nearly impossible cases. No one would know what to do in these situations."

S.N. "I think that what made them impossible was the behavior of the nurses and doctors. I think that they were afraid that they didn't know what to do."

S.N. "In the drama, Neoptolemus figures out what to do, and it is a simple thing to do, he tells the truth."

S.N. "Are you saying that if these patients had been told the truth they would have behaved differently?"

S.N. "Yes, I think that if people had said to this homeless man that they did not understand why he was so angry, things would have gone differently."

S.N.   "Maybe they would have with the woman on the respirator, too. But they would have to have been very patient with her, since she would have a lot of fear of being breathless."

S.N.   "But maybe Philoktetes wouldn't have agreed to leave the island initially if he had known the truth."

S.N.   "That lie caused Philoktetes a lot of suffering."

S.N.   "I want to point out that I do not understand the purpose of the Greek chorus. To me they seem to be like the echo of everyone. Sort of a group of people that make everyone feel okay to go ahead and do whatever it is they were going to do anyway, or want to do."

S.N.   "When Neoptolemus says that he sees Philoktetes and has pity for him, they jump in and express sympathy, too:

> *I pity him for all his woes,*
> *for his distress, for his loneliness,*
> *with no countryman at his side.*

(McNamee, p. 17)

S.N.   "They help Neoptolemus lie to Philoktetes at first by firing up the false notion that Neoptolemus hates Odysseus."

S.N.   "All of that was to get Philoktetes to feel sympathetic towards him."

S.N.   "But, let me remind you, Philoktetes is able to gain Neoptolemus' sympathy, also. He tells him how he was abandoned and how awful the 10 years have been."

S.N.   "Both men believe one another and Philoktetes begs to be taken back to Greece:

> *I am trying to kneel before you, a cripple,*
> *lame. Do not leave me in this lonely place.*

(McNamee, p. 30)

S.N.   "So, we have Philoktetes relieved that he is finally getting off the island. He's collecting his few belongings when all of a sudden he is overcome with pain in his wound."

S.N.   "It must have been one of those deep infections that keep erupting, his foot must have been terribly deformed."

S.N.   "He calls these episodes 'my sickness.'"

S.N.   "It's the kind of pain that is so bad, it does take over the whole person. He even says:

It sears through my blood!
I am destroyed! I am being devoured!

(McNamee, p. 41)

S.N.   "He begs Neoptolemus to cut off his foot!"

S.N.   "I have sympathy for Neoptolemus in the face of this kind of pain. Most of us wouldn't know what to do either. I would be afraid that I couldn't help. I know we all would feel awful that anyone had to suffer like that."

S.N.   "We would be afraid, you're right."

S.N.   "At least Neoptolemus asks what he should do."

S.N.   "And Philoktetes' reply is really what I think a lot of people in this same situation would like to say but can't:

Do not be afraid. Do not leave me.

(McNamee, p. 44)

S.N.   "You can see that Neoptolemus is having a change of heart, that he does not, can not, go on deceiving him:

I grieve for you sir. Your pain is mine.

(McNamee, p. 44)

S.N.   "Neoptolemus sees that Philoktetes has had a crisis, the infected foot has festered and erupted with pus and blood. He is so wasted by the severe pain that he falls asleep."

S.N.   "And once again, the chorus tries to persuade Neoptolemus that the time is ripe to make off with the bow, pretty much in the same vein as the day Odysseus first abandoned Philoktetes.

The man is blind and helpless now,
stretched out in the darkness—
he is master not of hand, not of foot, not of anything.

(McNamee, p. 47)

S.N.   "This is the part that moved me the most. This wounded man had been ignored, really forgotten for 10 long years. He lived all alone on this scruffy island with this rotten infection that never went away. He is so relieved to finally be rescued:

> *Blessed is the light that follows sleep,*
> *blessed is a friend's protection.*
> *These things are beyond my wildest hopes,*
> *that you would pity me and care for my sorrows*
> *that you would remain by me and endure my woes.*

(McNamee, p. 47, 48)

S.N.   "I know, and then Philoktetes senses that something has gone wrong after feeling this wonderful relief. And worse, he thinks he has made Neoptolemus sick because of his awful infection."

S.N.   "Well, to Neoptolemus' credit, he admits to his lie, really that he lied about everything."

S.N.   "Philoktetes was in a rage, he was betrayed by his own friend's son. And this is after he begged for his help."

S.N.   "It's no wonder that Philoktetes threatens to kill himself. He loses any hope he had of getting free of the island. And then he sees the man he hates the most, Odysseus."

S.N.   "Odysseus never wavers, he thinks he is justified in his actions right up to the end. He is stunned that Neoptolemus is not going to go along with him. He wants to capture Philoktetes and take him back by force."

S.N.   "Don't forget, Odysseus is the general of the Greek army and he has a war to fight."

S.N.   "In the face of that kind of pressure, I think that Neoptolemus is brave to defy his commander, to show loyalty to Philoktetes."

S.N.   "Odysseus believes he is 'a man who responds to occasion.' He tells Neoptolemus to let Philoktetes go, they don't need him because they have the magic bow, he thinks he can shoot it, himself."

S.N.   "This is the last straw for Philoktetes, now they are going to desert him and they are taking the one means he has of getting food for himself."

S.N.   "Would you trust someone who had done this kind of thing to you?"

S.N.   "I can't let this pass by, this time, in the drama, the chorus almost blames Philoktetes for his own mess when he gives up hope of getting off Lemnos.

> *You brought this on yourself, unbending man,*
> *You could have found a way out*
> *when it was possible to make a sensible choice,*
> *but you took the worse over the better fate.*

(McNamee, p. 59)

S.N.   "They do beg him to set aside his hatreds."

S.N.   "This is just exactly like the situation I told you all about earlier. Remember the homeless man who had burned his feet so badly? Well, in this case, the chorus and Odysseus are just like the doctors and the nurses blaming the man for his own wounds, saying he brought it on himself. They hatch a plan to get him to leave the hospital because they can't stand him but they know he needs the kind of care he's getting there. They essentially toss him out, blame him for it because he caused his own wounds, and his homelessness, and then they blame him for not coming up with the solution to the whole mess!"

S.N.   "I remember seeing that man's face that day. He was huddled over in his rattlely old wheelchair. The nurses had gotten him some clean, second-hand clothes and a coat from storage. It all was too big for him, he was so thin. He was trying to wheel himself down the hall as quickly as possible. He was so angry but he was embarrassed at the same time. I felt just awful, and helpless, too."

S.N.   "No one had anything to say, everybody just seemed relieved not to have to deal with him anymore. I kept thinking about what happened, over and over. I tried to think of a different ending to that story. This play had some possible answers, but Heracles is not going to appear on any hospital unit. And no one that day on the nursing or medical staff defied that senior resident who threw him out. It was like getting a dishonorable discharge from the service or something."

S.N. "It makes me wonder what would have happened if someone had challenged that doctor by way of admitting to the homeless man that the staff couldn't figure out how to help him but they wanted to try."

S.N. "Whoever did that would have to be prepared for a lot of anger from him."

S.N. "Who? The doctor or the patient?"

S.N. "Maybe both. It would take a lot of guts, I know that."

S.N. "The amazing thing is that nobody kept their dignity the way that it turned out. The man was humiliated and hurt, the staff could hardly be proud of their actions, or should I say inaction."

S.N. "It wasn't just Heracles showing up that saved Philoktetes. I think he was taken back when Neoptolemus told him the truth and gave him back his bow, defying Odysseus. And, I think that he believed Neoptolemus when he told him he wished for him to be cared for and to 'give up his anguish.'"

S.N. "I believe you are right. Somehow he suspected what it cost Neoptolemus to admit his wrong doing. Maybe he saw his real desire to help. But his admission also allowed Philoktetes to keep his dignity. I mean, if you apologize to someone, that shows respect for that person."

S.N. "And then, because of that, I think, Philoktetes can let go of his bitterness and anger. He does, in a sense, surrender his hatreds and is then able to accept the offered rescue from that lonely island."

S.N. "You know, one of the major reasons why Neoptolemus is able to admit his deed is because he realizes that his lie will not only hurt Philoktetes very badly, but also, that it will hurt him. I mean, he has enough character, even though he is very young, to know that he will always be bothered, the rest of his life, if he betrays this sick man."

S.N. "That's what will always bother me . . . I couldn't figure out what to do for the homeless man."

S.N. "He might have been like Philoktetes, it might have been tough to get him to accept the help he needed. Maybe too many things had already happened to him, too."

S.N. "And, don't forget, it's possible that his hatred of everyone keeps him going, just like Philoktetes' did. If Philoktetes

hadn't had all that bitterness and hatred of Odysseus he probably wouldn't have survived those 10 long years."

S.N.   "You are missing an important fact . . . what happened to
both of these men, being cast out of society, exiled, really,
when you think of it, should never have happened in the first
place."

S.N.   "It's a kind of indictment against both societies, isn't it?"

S.N.   "Well, it is a known fact that a society's morality is reflected
in the way it cares for the sick and the poor."

CONCLUSION

Campbell, the distinguished Classics Professor of St. Andrews,
explained why the study of Greek tragedy is so potent and lasting.

> In a great community there is a mass of grief and care which in
> the common daylight of the marketplace and the assembly is
> conveniently ignored. Thus each heart is left to a knowledge of
> its own bitterness, and pines in isolation. But when men are
> drawn together to a spectacle of imagined woe, placed vividly
> before the eye, the fountain of tears within them is unlocked,
> and a society of grief is gained without confession. Feeling is at
> once consoled by communion, and sheltered in the privacy of a
> crowd. For all who have any depth in them, however habitually
> light-hearted, such an occasional overflow is tranquillizing,
> while those whose burden presses heavily are eased and com-
> forted. They are rapt from the narrow contemplation of their
> own destiny into a world where all private trouble is annihi-
> lated and yet is typified so as to give an excuse for tears.
>
> *(Campbell, 1880, p. 22)*

There is a continuing relevance to Sophocles' portrayal of the
wounded Philoktetes' suffering in exile, betrayed by his own people. His plight is echoed today in our own society that cannot always come to terms compassionately with the sick and disfigured.
Thus, it is an awareness of this burden and its sequelae that nursing
must struggle to achieve. As the last student said, ". . . a society's
morality is reflected in the way it cares for the sick and the poor."

Real sorrow was expressed by this class for the ancient Greek, Sophoclean figure, and direct analogies to contemporary men and women were easily made. Most importantly, a closer look at the just action that can occur when veracity is honored is especially relevant. The sick and the poor are too wounded to find solutions to their plight. And their plight is worsened beyond endurance by those in a position to alleviate their suffering but who cannot act out of fear or ignorance, and those who deceive "for their own greater good."

Following are student stories written in response to the Philoctetean theme of the willful abandonment of individuals in need of care and concern. They convey a fresh understanding of the implications of the suffering caused by this exile and the cost to the nurse who chooses to transcend personal reasons for not acting.

IRENE
by Terry McCauley

"I-I-I-wa-wa-wa-," Irene's fragile twig fingers reached out hopefully, emphasizing her struggle to get the nurse's attention.

"What is it?", the nurse demanded, pausing impatiently outside of Irene's door. "D-D-D-Do- yo-y-y-," Irene groped for words.

"Look, Irene, I'm busy. I *do not* have time for your whining." The nurse continued on down the hall. A high pitched wail of anger, hurt, and frustration followed.

"God, what a pain in the ass," the nurse said to nobody in particular as she began grabbing clean sheets out of the linen closet.

This was just another hazy, humid afternoon at the Community Nursing Home, and the sound of Irene's screaming ruptured the air, sending the birds that had been merrily singing outside her window off in a flutter of wings.

I had been working at the nursing home since June, and Irene's outbursts had become a part of the daily routine, and no longer startled me, as they did the birds. Irene was a small delicate woman, whose coke bottle glasses made her soft puppy-like eyes seem comically enormous in her shrunken face. In fact, she reminded me of those puppies that are often pictured on little kid's puzzles, with the sad eyes and droopy ears. No longer able to walk (I could not imagine those ribbon legs bearing any weight) Irene depended on staff to move her from bed to chair and bathroom and often much to her shame, when we went in to conduct rounds or bring her to supper, her bed was soiled. Irene's mental faculties were deceptively intact. However, she could not speak in anything but a stuttering whine, and few had the patience to allow her to complete a sentence. For hours she would sit in the doorway of her room, hen-like claws pecking randomly at passing staff, pleading for recognition.

Her screaming climaxed and died out, but now the light over her door blinked importantly. I walked in and turned it off.

"What is it Irene? Do you have to use the bathroom?"

"Y-Y-Yes." A flicker of relief passed over her face, and her cheeks flushed as she bobbed her white curls up and down.

I lifted her from the bed and placed her in her wheelchair, and carted her over to the bathroom. When she was through, I wheeled her in her chair to sit by the door.

"C-C-C-Cold."

I looked down at her plaid dress that buttoned down the front. Lunch's applesauce was drying nicely on the slip that showed beneath. I selected a pretty green sweater from her closet.

"I like this one. Do you, Irene?"

"Y-Yes."

I put the sweater gently around her hunched shoulders. I had an impulsive urge to hug her frail scrap of a body. I didn't. I was in a hurry.

Nine o'clock finally arrived, and I noted with some satisfaction that all of my assigned patients were safely tucked away for the night, and I could relax for a moment.

A light on the panel went on.

"C-C-Come, c-c-come!" Irene's whine pierced my moment.

"Oh, Irene, STOP! YOU'RE FINE!" the nurse exploded.

"N-N-No, c-come!"

"Go to SLEEP! . . . She had better not be like this all night, because I can't take it." Wild hand gestures emphasized her point, as the nurse searched frantically about the desk for a misplaced medication sheet.

"P-Please!" Her whine was desperate and hopeless.

"I'm not going," an aide said defiantly as she plunked herself down at the nurses' station. "She's not my patient."

"I'll go." My conscience was gnawing, and after all, Irene's bed was right next to the nurses' station.

"Yes, Irene?" I asked.

"H-H-Hot."

I flicked on the light and illuminated the room. Without her glasses on, her eyes looked small and empty. She lay like a rag doll beneath the covers, the only signs of life being in her eyes, and a small lipless mouth forming silent "ohs."

"Can't you make up your mind?" I chided gently and smiled a little.

She said nothing, but a whisper of a smile revealed dry pink gums. My smile broadened, became genuine, as I pulled back the top cover.

"Are you comfy now?"

"Y-Y-Yes."

"Okay. Goodnight."

"W-W-Wait!" Although I had turned off the light, I could imagine those spidery fingers groping, pleading in the darkness.

"No, I said goodnight. I'll see you tomorrow." I closed the door, sighed and walked back to the nurses' station. Cries of indignation followed in my wake. Three days later Irene was dead.

Today, when I think of Irene, I feel a strong sense of shame and remorse. To acknowledge suffering and provide empathy is an act of compassion. To acknowledge suffering and then ignore it is heartless. Irene's suffering was like that of Philoktetes, whose suffering was also ignored. Philoktetes suffered unbearably, and without pity or compassion. He was stranded on the island alone, and when it looked as though he was going to find truth and justice through Neoptolemus, he was deceived once more, and cast into the depths of despair and suffering. He had no compassion, no justice, and therefore, no hope.

Like Philoktete's, Irene's suffering was never justly ameliorated. She died a miserable, hopeless human being. She died alone without compassion or peace. Irene was trapped in her body, Philoktetes was trapped on the island. Her stuttering was a barrier that no one cared to break through, and the pain and frustration that this caused her must have been nearly intolerable. Those desperate pleading eyes and her tentative wisps of fingers said more than words could, and they too, were ignored. The episodic, infrequent displays of compassion shown Irene were most often generated out of guilt, and therefore were not really compassionate acts at all, and little hope could be garnered from them. As Philoktetes was deceived, Irene was confronted with deception everyday. A staff member showing a momentary display of compassion would nurture a tiny seedling of hope, of truth, of worth, only to be crushed in the next moment with a cruel "Shut up, Irene!" Again and again Irene glimpsed hope, and again and again it was stamped out.

The Difficult Patient
by Stacey Cordwell

"Oh, you have Mr. Brown. He's a very difficult patient—very hard to handle," the charge nurse said to the student nurse, rolling her eyes.

"Good luck. He's ninety-nine years old, blind, almost completely deaf, incontinent of everything, and totally out of it. You've got to practically yell into his right ear if you expect him to hear anything. And be careful when you give him a bed bath because he likes to punch and kick nurses," she added somewhat haughtily.

To an observer peering into Room 288, two things would be startlingly obvious; the ghostly, emaciated old man, and the frightened, pale student nurse. His motionless body contrasted vividly with her trembling hands. She repeatedly glanced at the sleeping man as she hurried around the room getting items ready for his bed bath. She didn't approach Mr. Brown, there seemed to be an invisible barrier around him.

A tall, impeccably dressed doctor entered the room to examine Mr. Brown. The student intently watched his interaction with the man. As the doctor leaned over toward Mr. Brown's right ear, the student also leaned. Suddenly, the doctor bellowed, "Hey, Mr. Brown! Wake up!" Startled, the student stepped back and watched Mr. Brown's struggle to turn his frail body away from the intrusion. He curled up into a fetal position, wrapping his arthritic hands tightly around his legs. The young nurse glared at the doctor in disbelief. With fire in her eyes, she walked briskly out of the room. Pacing the hall, waiting until the doctor left, she tried to rid her mind of the insensitivity that she had just witnessed.

When she returned to Mr. Brown, she found him stretched out on his back, chest bare, perfectly still except for the irregular, labored breathing. The student took a deep breath and walked to him with assurance. Feeling tentative for a second, she placed her hand gently over his before leaning near his ear to speak to him. Her eyes widened with surprise when Mr. Brown squeezed her hand in response. She grinned when the corners of his mouth turned up ever so slightly. Continuing with the morning routine, the student lightly touched his hand each time she spoke to him. He cooperated fully during his bed bath.

Bath completed, he timidly sought out her hand once more just as the charge nurse passed by the doorway, a puzzled expression on her face. The student glanced up and smiled contentedly.

You're Welcome
by Jill Cooper

I heard the stretcher being wheeled into the room as one of the nurses shouted, "Jill, we need a set up in Room 8!" I immediately went into the room to get things prepared for suturing. As I was hustling about I introduced myself and greeted the patient in the usual manner. "Hi! What happened?" I asked. I got only a few incoherent grunts for a response. I turned to get another look at the patient. He was about sixty-five, I thought. His arms were contorted and shaking uncontrollably. I went outside the room to where the doctor was reading his medical record. "Cerebral Palsy," she said, "I'm going to need a lot of help with this one."

She entered the room to examine the man's hand. There was a deep two inch laceration at the base of the thumb and it was still bleeding. "This will be quick," she mumbled to me. "Just hold down the hand." I attempted to press the man's hand against the arm board. It was difficult to manuever to the right position because of his awkward, shaking arm which had been deformed by his palsy. "We're going to fix the cut on your thumb," I said to Mr. Wood. The doctor was trying to manuever his arm on the board. I could tell that she was getting aggravated with the awkwardness of it all. Finally, she found a position and said, "Here—like this," and I grasped his arm as she showed me.

Systematically, the doctor prepared the syringe and wordlessly began to inject the contents. Quickly, I said to the man, "Just a little medicine to make it numb. This is the worst part." I could tell by his grunts and rocking of his head that he was very agitated. The doctor glanced up from her work to look at me. She chuckled and said, "It makes no difference to him." I was caught off guard by her indifference.

I continued to talk to Mr. Wood throughout the procedure, all the while feeling that the doctor thought me foolish. Each time I explained a part of the procedure, I thought I saw a mocking, disapproving smirk at the corner of her lips. I felt extremely self-conscious and insecure with every word I said. I wondered if it was even worth it, after all. My explanation was received with only a kind of grunt from Mr. Wood. I had no idea whether or not he understood a word I was saying, but with the possibility that he could hear and comprehend (which I hoped was possible), I continued.

When the suturing was complete, I put a dressing on the wound and informed him that he had gotten eight stitches. Then I called the ambulance service and asked them to come for Mr. Wood. I followed that call with one to the nursing home informing them that Mr. Wood would be returning shortly from the emergency room. Looking at Mr. Wood, I suggested that he relax, someone would be coming soon to take him back.

I proceeded to clean the area and ready the room for the next patient when I heard him grunting again. I turned to see his head lifted off the pillow, turned slightly in my direction. I watched, wondering what all of this straining was about. Then, with his wounded hand raised up, he formed words that, though they were very slurred, were vivid to me . . . "Thank you."

The Exile of Illness: Tolstoi, *The Death of Ivan Ilych*

4

Art is a means of union among men, joining them together in the same feelings, and (is) indispensable for the life and progress towards well-being of individuals and of humanity.

Leo Tolstoi

CLASS DISCUSSION

Students closely read and annotated this novella prior to class meeting. The class concentrated on four central themes: Ivan Ilych's funeral; his childhood, young adult years and his marriage to Praskovya and their subsequent children; Ivan's wound and illness including interactions with health care professionals, family, colleagues, and Gerasim; and mortality and the soul. These thematic discussions are recorded here. Guided by the annotations written in

Portions of the précis appeared in *Clinical Nurse Specialist* and in a research presentation in the "National Nursing Conference on Leadership: Moving Towards the Future, New Ideas, New Directions," at the University of Michigan, September 1986.

THE DEATH OF IVAN ILYCH

Leo Tolstoi. (1886) Translated by Alymer Maud (1960) New York:
New American Library. By permission of Oxford University Press,
Inc.

Characters of the Novella

The Golovina Family Household
Ivan Ilych Golovina
Praskovya Fëdorovna Golovina, his wife
Vladimir Ivanich, their son, "Volodya"
Lisa, their daughter
Fëdor Petrovich, their daughter's fiancé
Gerasim, household "serf" and carer of Ivan Ilych in his illness
Peter, the footman
Law Colleagues of Ivan Ilych
Ivan Egorovich Shebek
Fëdor Vasilievich
Peter Ivanovich
Mikhail Mikhalovich
Swartz
The Doctors
Leshchetitsky, a specialist
Michael Danilovich, the Golovina's regular doctor

THE DEATH OF IVAN ILYCH illustrates the despair and isolation
of a dying man in the middle-class society of 19th century Russia. It

(*Continued on page 74.*)

their personal copies of the novella, students quoted directly from this text when illustrating a point, discussing a character's behavior or making analogies to contemporary issues and stories. Note the depth and variety of the responses as they unfold.

THE FUNERAL

S.N.   "I feel like I just attended the funeral myself after reading this!"

S.N.   "Me too! I feel just like I was there and it wasn't pleasant. I am surprised Tolstoi started out the novella with the funeral. You sort of think funerals should go at the end, not the beginning."

S.N.   "I am going to admit that I have sympathy for his friends who tried to get out of going."

S.N.   "I don't have much sympathy for them. They remind me of the men in the Citizen's Bureau in *Ikiru*. They were angling to see which one would get his job when he was gone."

S.N.   "Also, they thought how irritating it was to have to go to Ivan's wake."

S.N.   "It's worse than that because they all knew that he was fatally ill but they learned about his death in the newspaper. That means that they hadn't been to see him for quite awhile."

S.N.   "That is similar to the men in *Ikiru* who knew that he was ill, he wasn't showing up for work, yet no one went to look for him or anything."

S.N.   "That's not surprising in *Ikiru*, they weren't close anyhow."

S.N.   "But it is surprising in this story because Ivan played bridge and had dinner with these guys all of the time."

S.N.   "Maybe they were worried about what would be asked of them?"

S.N.   "Well, they did wonder about the widow's financial status."

S.N.   "I think that they were just glad that they were alive. Remember, each one thought, or felt, thankfully, 'Well, he's dead, but I'm alive!'" (Tolstoi, 1960, p. 97)

S.N.   "That's natural enough, I would have the same reaction myself."

specifically explores the deep moral and spiritual suffering of a lawyer and bureaucrat, Ivan Ilych, as he searches in his final illness for the meaning of his life. As readers face the knowledge of impending death with Ivan Ilych and his family and colleagues, they witness the need for truth and the compassion of forgiveness. Though completed 100 years ago, the themes of this short, crystalline novel are familiar today in a world that honors promotion and gratification of the self before the interest of others. Tolstoi's rounded view of Ivan's world and intimate knowledge of his personal suffering provide a deeper understanding of the pain of loss and the hope that compassion creates (Young-Mason, 1988, p. 180)

"Ivan Ilych's life had been most simple and ordinary and therefore most terrible" (Tolstoi, p. 104), and as Tolstoi reveals the vignettes of Ivan's "ordinary" life, the reader begins to understand its terribleness. For it seems that "in law school he was just what he remained for the rest of his life, a capable, cheerful, good-natured and social man, though strict in the fulfillment of what he considered his duty: and he considered his duty to be what was so considered by those in authority" (Tolstoi, p. 105). He was always attracted to those people in higher station and emulated their talk, manners, and politics without any desire to be different.

Upon graduation from law school and with the very best of furnishings, Ivan set out for his first position, secured by his father, as aide to the provincial governor. Once settled in his new surroundings he arranged an easy, agreeable life. He performed his official tasks punctually and thoroughly and at the same time amused himself pleasantly and decorously. He had affairs and carousals, but we are told all this was done with "clean hands, in clean linen, with French phrases and above all among people of the best society and consequently with the approval of people of rank" (Tolstoi, p. 106).

When reforms came to the judicial institutions with the emancipation of the serfs (in 1861), Ivan was offered a post as examining

(Continued on page 76.)

S.N.   "The behavior of his friend, Swartz, and others at the wake was a bit surprising. Well, maybe not when you think of what we have already said. I guess it wouldn't be too unusual to find some joking and a serious wish for it to be over as quickly as possible."

S.N.   "I know, but, I was at a wake last week. It was in a funeral home and the body was there for all to see, the casket lid was open. You could, very clearly, see his face. I can tell you, I didn't know any more than Swartz did, what I should do."

S.N.   "The same things could be said of Praskovya, Ivan's wife. I don't think she acted entirely appropriately either. She gets his friend, Peter Ivanovich, into the drawing room and begins to tell him, in detail, how Ivan suffered. She makes it sound like he should have pity for her because of her suffering, instead of for his dead friend."

S.N.   "It seems like she was doing this to get more money from the government through Peter."

S.N.   "Here, then, is another example of a person telling 'the truth' for personal gain."

S.N.   "She sounds like a martyr to me. I'd have a hard time with her."

S.N.   "But you can't blame her! She is a widow and she needs money to live on."

S.N.   "Wait! Listen to what she is saying:

> He suffered terribly the last few days. Oh, terribly! He screamed unceasingly, not for minutes but for hours. For the last three days he screamed incessantly. It was unbearable. It was unendurable. I cannot understand how I bore it; you could hear him three rooms off. Oh, what I have suffered.
>
> *(Tolstoi, 1960, p. 101)*

S.N.   "She, flat out, says, 'Oh, what I have suffered.'" (Tolstoi, 1960, p. 101)

S.N.   "But relatives *do* suffer when a loved one is sick and in a lot of pain."

S.N.   "I don't think she felt that bad . . . she was pretty superficial and there is plenty of evidence for my saying that."

magistrate in another province. In his new position, he conducted his duties in the same "*comme il faut*" way (Tolstoi, p. 107), inspiring mediocre if general respect. Many people were dependent upon him, he had power to call any official before him, power which he never abused, although he enjoyed thinking of it proudly and, in fact, it was the chief attraction of this new position.

It was in this circle that he met his future bride, Praskovya Fëderovna, a young girl of a good family, property, and decent appearance. Ivan calculated that he might try to make a better match, but here was a nice, correct girl who had an inheritance and who sympathized with his views, and whom his colleagues thought an appropriate match, *comme il faut*, and so they were married.

At first, life seemed agreeable with new furniture, linens, dishes, and amorous moments. Ivan believed the marriage would not interfere with his decorous life, but then his wife became pregnant. She began to upset this even life by becoming jealous without reason, demanding his full devotion. Initially, Ivan tried to ignore this unpleasant occurrence and live life as before, but Praskovya became relentless in her demands until he submitted to her. Alarmed, Ivan attempted to assert his independence from his wife by becoming engrossed in official duties and appointments. When the child came and difficulties ensued involving feedings and illnesses, Ivan's "official" boundaries were thus already in place.

Seventeen years passed during which he was promoted to public prosecutor. Three of their five children died and by degrees family life became more unpleasant. But to outward appearances all was comme il faut. If this ordinary propriety was challenged, Ivan continued to retreat to official duties, bridge games, and collegial dinners.

When Ivan was passed over for a promotion he desired, he despaired for the first time in his life. Disconsolate, he took his family to the country for the entire summer, unable to bear his angry and bitter feelings. At his brother-in-law's house, things became impossible

(*Continued on page 78.*)

S.N.   "She scared his friend plenty, listen to what he's thinking:

> The thought of the sufferings of this man he had
> known so intimately, first as a merry school boy, then
> as a school-mate, and later as a grown-up colleague;
> suddenly struck Peter Ivanovich with horror, despite an
> unpleasant consciousness of his own and this woman's
> dissimulation. He again saw that brow and that nose
> pressing down on the lip, and felt afraid for himself.
>
> *(Tolstoi, 1960, pp. 101, 102)*

S.N.   "His usual behavior takes over though, I don't think he can
stand unpleasant thoughts very long. He thinks:

> Three days of frightful suffering and then death. Why,
> that might suddenly, at any time, happen to me.
>
> *(Tolstoi, 1960, p. 102)*

"But then thinks, this happened to Ivan, not me. Also, if he
continued to think about it he would be 'yielding to depression.' And depression was to be avoided."

S.N.   "I think that is a natural thought, too. It *is* depressing to go
to a wake or funeral. You have to keep your spirits up, don't
you? Otherwise you imagine all sorts of gloomy things."

S.N.   "Yes, like imagining how the person died, what they were
thinking about when they were dying, whether they were in a
lot of pain."

S.N.   "And, what is it like to know for certain that you are going to
die? How scary is it?"

S.N.   "There are bigger issues, too. Such as, did he believe in an
after-life? Did he think that this life, the life he lived was it?
Did he think that when he was dead, that was it? Nothing
more?"

S.N.   "This is all very upsetting, and in a way more so than when
we saw *Ikiru* because though we got attached to Watanabe, I
didn't feel as bad at his wake as I did when I read this."

S.N.   "Oh, I think that the sight of Watanabe, the night he died,
sitting in that swing, in the dark, all alone, singing, is incredibly sad."

and he struck out for St. Petersburg, desperate for any change, willing to take any post, anywhere, so long as it offered more money. By sheer luck, on the train to St. Petersburg, a colleague told him of a possible position within the courts. He was fortunate to secure the appointment and thrilled at the increase in salary it granted him. Enormously relieved, he threw himself into preparing a home for his family, *comme il faut*, by buying antiques, arranging furniture, picking out wallpaper, hanging curtains. It was during one such episode that he fell from a ladder and deeply bruised his side, an accident which eventually took his life. The home, when completed, resembled all other homes of the middle class who wanted to appear rich.

For a time life flowed along in the new home; the couple had declared a truce, and there was a new social circle to cultivate. Their daughter became popular and there was talk of an engagement to a "correct" young man, the son of a prominent lawyer.

Then, Ivan began to experience symptoms of his own mortality in the form of a queer taste in his mouth and discomfort in his side from his injury. Praskovya challenged Ivan to do something about his health. The physician involved treated Ivan in the same detached, authoritarian manner with which Ivan himself had treated the accused in his courtroom, gave him a probable cause for his discomfort pending a further diagnostic study of his urine, and dismissed him. Ivan felt set aside, a mere nuisance. When he pressed the physician as to the seriousness of his symptoms, the latter became condescending. And, sadly, when he then attempted to explain his condition to his wife and daughter, they, too, brushed him aside.

Ivan tried to convince himself that it was not so serious and denied his symptoms, but every family dispute, every bad bridge hand, intensified his discomfort. Once he tried to master these situations; now he unleashed his anger at events and began reading medical texts and consulting other doctors. Those consulted recommended contradictory therapies.

(*Continued on page 80.*)

S.N.   "But this novella makes you feel bad every step of the way. I know what Ivan was thinking, how scared he was, and worst of all, how lonely he was."

S.N.   "Yes, but how can you measure such things. One found out what would give meaning to his life months before he died. The other found out hours before he died. So, in a way, it seems like Ivan was tormented longer, for months and months."

S.N.   "This all really makes me wonder what patients are thinking that we take care of. I was a home health aide this past summer and most of my people were elderly and chronically ill. They were alone for hours and hours everyday. And when I think of that, the loneliness, it seems worse than some of the physical pain they suffered."

S.N.   "That all depends on how bad the physical pain was, if it kept them immobilized."

S.N.   "Well, if they suffered from the kinds of remembering that Ivan did, they might not have been able to overcome any pain they had. Emotional pain is debilitating, too."

FAMILIAL LIFE OF AN ORDINARY MAN

S.N.   "Ivan Ilych is one of those people who never had to suffer much to get an education or a job. He was a spoiled kid. One of his brothers was not successful in school and the family just let him drift away."

S.N.   "I read that when he graduated from law school, his father, who was a civil servant, found him his first position."

S.N.   "But he was a lawyer and better educated than his brothers or sister."

S.N.   "It was natural that he get a good position."

S.N.   "Well, I am struck with the opening sentence here; 'Ivan Ilych's life had been most simple and most ordinary and therefore most terrible.'" (Tolstoi, 1960, p. 104)

S.N.   "If his colleagues had the same beginnings, it's no wonder that they were considered ordinary, too."

As the pain in his side grew more severe and his breath became foul, he lost appetite and strength and was no longer able to deceive himself. He knew something was terribly wrong, but neither his wife, family, nor colleagues acknowledged his disease. His wife's self-pity intensified and with it her anger. She blamed his illness and irritability on him, seeing him as a nuisance, an obstacle to her and her daughter's social enjoyment.

In the law courts he saw that his colleagues were watching him carefully, waiting for him to vacate his post. His friends joshed him about his low spirits, trivializing his pain and despair. Isolated by the anger, blame, and denial of those around him, Ivan was in torment, on the brink of an abyss. The awareness of the torment, the sense of loneliness, and the physical pain petrified and mystified him. Inwardly, he wondered where would he go if he died. "When I am not, what will there be? There will be nothing. Then where shall I be when I am not anymore? Can this be dying? No, I don't want to!" (Tolstoi, p. 130–131). He feared his death and hated his family for continuing their lives.

During the third month of his illness, his suffering was his only preoccupation. He was heavily sedated and needed constant help with physical care and habits. Gerasim, his young servant, performed all these unpleasant tasks calmly and with dignity, sparing his master any possible embarrassment. He, alone, was able to bear the truth with Ivan, that he was dying and needed every comfort and sat for hours holding up the suffering man's legs because that was the only position in which Ivan could find relief. Gerasim's presence was the only one that brought peace.

In the last weeks of his life, Ivan Ilych was medicated always and was thus somewhat stupefied. He had a distinct feeling of being pushed into a narrow black sack, which he wished for but feared. In his terrible loneliness he wept openly for himself because of his "helplessness, his terrible loneliness, the cruelty of man, the cruelty

(*Continued on page 82.*)

S.N.   "Here is a clue to what Tolstoi meant by ordinary, and that is someone who goes along with the norm, doesn't think for himself."

> In law school he was just what he remained for the rest of his life, a capable, cheerful, good-natured and social man, though strict in the fulfillment of what he considered his duty; and he considered his duty to be what was so considered by those in authority. In fact, he was always attracted to people in higher station and emulated their talk, manners, and politics without any desire to be different.
>
> *(Young-Mason, 1988, p. 181)*

S.N.   "He might have been a cad, in a way."
S.N.   "Why on earth do you say that?"
S.N.   "He always had it just the way he wanted it and this goes for his love life, too."
S.N.   "How is that?"
S.N.   "Listen to this. He had affairs, lots of affairs, and these affairs were conducted

> with clean hands, with French phrases and above all among people of the best society and consequently with approval of people of rank.
>
> *(Tolstoi, 1960, p. 106)*

S.N.   "He doesn't have much of a back bone if he can only do things if his superiors approve of them."

S.N.   "Here is a good example of what I mean about his love life. He had just the right position, and he has all of these affairs. He's happy. Then he meets Praskovya at a dinner dance. He can see that she likes him a lot. He has no intention of marrying, but when she falls in love with him, he thinks, 'Really, why shouldn't I marry?'"

S.N.   "Yes, here's how he reasons it out: She isn't bad looking, she comes from a good family, she has a little property. Maybe I could make a more brilliant match, but this is a good one."

of God, and the absence of God" (Tolstoi, p. 146). His inner dialogue with God intensified with his pain and despair. He realized his wish to live as he did before his illness was a hollow one, because as he reviewed his life he recollected with horror that after childhood there was little joy, love, or friendship. His marriage seemed a mere accident, a disenchantment in a false society, a mere push for higher wages, a hollow memory. Could it be that his life had been senseless, even horrible? How, when he did everything so properly? He could not justify or come to terms with himself and realized there was nothing to defend. He began to wonder how he could rectify the fact of losing all that was given him (Tolstoi, p. 148, paraphrased).

During the last three days of his life, his painful search for meaning in his life became unbearable and his physical pain excruciating. His self-doubt unresolved, he knew his death was near. While he wanted to end his agonies, he was restrained by the wish to believe that his life had been a good one. At this moment he was struck with a force in his chest that made him breathless. He thought, "Yes, it was all not the right thing, but, that's no matter. It can be done, but what is the right thing?" (Tolstoi, p. 154–155). At this precise moment he reached out to his son who seized his father's hand and pressed it to his lips crying. Ivan saw that his son Vasya was stricken with sorrow at losing his father. This knowledge awakened in him a sensitivity to another's suffering. He realized that his family was suffering too and that he must forgive and release them in order to release himself. His despair for himself and anger toward his family disappeared and he was able to transcend his physical pain. In place of death, he saw light (Tolstoi, p. 156, paraphrased).

S.N.   "He also gets the approval, once again, of his associates."

S.N.   "You are all talking about him as though he were a bad man—but he wasn't. In the story we see him as a magistrate. We also see that he likes to flaunt his authority a bit, he likes the fact that people are a bit nervous waiting to see him. But, we also learn:

> Ivan Ilych never abused his power; he tried on the contrary to soften its expression, but the consciousness of it and of the possibility of softening its effect, supplied the chief interest and attraction of his office.
>
> *(Tolstoi, 1960, p. 107)*

S.N.   "Here is a point that I want to make because I think it is very important to know that a lawyer can think like this:

> In his work itself, especially in his examinations, he very soon acquired a method of eliminating all considerations irrelevant to the legal aspect of the case, and reducing even the most complicated case to a form in which it would be presented on paper only in its externals, completely excluding his personal opinion of the matter, while above all observing every prescribed formality.
>
> *(Tolstoi, 1960, pp. 107, 108)*

This is important because it tells me that he was stripping down the cases before him of the human element, either his or that of the person before him. It wouldn't feel real, it would make everyone some sort of reading out of a law book, a theory or something. I wouldn't have liked to come before him."

S.N.   "Some doctors and nurses think like this, too. It's dangerous, reducing the person to lab values and diagnostic test results, or behavioral norms."

S.N.   "Still, I do not believe he was a bad man."

S.N.   "I want to talk about the marriage because what happened to the Golovinas could happen to anyone."

S.N.   "I agree, I know a couple back home just like Ivan and Praskovya when they first married."

S.N.   "How could they be the same?"

S.N.   "Well, they had this big wedding and got all sorts of nice presents. They even got a house in the suburbs. I thought they had the ideal life. Then the wife charged all kinds of things for the house that they couldn't afford to pay for on the husband's salary."

S.N.   "That isn't exactly what happened here because it wasn't until Praskovya got pregnant that they started fighting."

S.N.   "I personally think that their marriage began in trouble. He married her because it was the right thing to do. Also, he thought that the marriage wouldn't interfere with the way he already lived his life."

S.N.   "Obviously he wasn't prepared to change much, so when Praskovya became pregnant and wanted more attention, he must have been surprised."

S.N.   "You are too kind. Sure she got demanding, and jealous of all the time he spent with his friends. But his reaction was to get busier at work."

S.N.   "So we shouldn't be surprised that the demands that the baby made on them didn't bring them together."

S.N.   "No, the baby didn't bring them together. And sad to say, they had five children in those 17 years and three of them died. Yet, nowhere in the story do you hear mentioned any shared sorrow for the lost babies."

S.N.   "True, and by degrees their marriage disintegrated."

S.N.   "But, yet, to all outward appearances it was 'comme il faut.'"

S.N.   "And Ivan just retreated to his official duties and bridge games and dinners with his cronies."

S.N.   "Okay, who took French? What does 'comme il faut' mean?"

S.N.   "I think it means something like 'as things should be,' you know, as everybody expects thing to be, like everybody else."

S.N.   "I noticed that nothing is mentioned about how they felt when they lost three babies."

S.N.   "They were really just leading two separate lives in the same house."

S.N.   "There are hints of awful quarrels and times when they didn't speak to one another."

S.N.   "They fought over the education of their son and Ivan was totally occupied with law. He even had other people to their home so that he wouldn't be alone with his wife."

S.N.   "I have a lot of sympathy for Praskovya because I think she was alone an awful lot and, also, because, in the beginning, she loved him and he didn't love her."

S.N.   "I think she got a bad deal."

S.N.   "No wonder she was so cranky all of the time, she felt betrayed."

S.N.   "I will admit that, when I read that Ivan was passed over for a promotion, I didn't feel too bad for him. I sort of felt that he deserved it."

S.N.   "That was the first time he ever felt depressed, and that's a wonder because he was well into his forties by then."

S.N.   "Yes, you'd think he would have been depressed about his home life."

S.N.   "He got depressed this time because he lost his temper for the first time at the office and people acted cold toward him. Even his father wouldn't help him out."

S.N.   "Just like the young couple I described in the suburbs, Ivan and Praskovya were living beyond their means, and that spells trouble."

S.N.   "He lucked out and ended up with a better position for more money."

S.N.   "It seems that way, but it was also the beginning of the end for him."

S.N.   "I don't see why you say that."

THE WOUND AND THE ILLNESS

S.N.   "Did you notice that Ivan Ilych gets carried away with his new position and the fact that he is earning more money? He travels alone to Petersberg to arrange the house. He redecorates the whole thing without his wife."

S.N.   "That is not surprising since they weren't together on any issue anyway."

S.N.   "This is when it happened. He rushes about buying new furniture, dishes, everything. He is trying to make the house look like those of the rich. He bangs his side very hard in a fall while trying to hang drapes by himself."

S.N.   "And that's the beginning of the end for Ivan."

S.N.   "Here's an irony, the house ends up looking just like all of the others."

S.N.   "I don't understand what he actually developed. Was it cancer?"

S.N.   "I think so and it must have been a deep bruise. It developed quickly because he has symptoms that begin within weeks, and then just get worse."

S.N.   "What were the symptoms?"

S.N.   "They began with something that doesn't seem reportable;

> Ivan Ilych sometimes said that he had a queer taste in his mouth and felt some discomfort in his side.
>
> *(Tolstoi, 1960, p. 120)*

S.N.   "But then it quickly developed along with psychological symptoms:

> But this discomfort increased and, though not exactly painful grew into a sense of pressure in his side accompanied by ill humor. And his irritability became worse and worse and began to mar the agreeable, easy and correct life that had been established in the Golovina family.
>
> *(Tolstoi, 1960, p. 120)*

S.N.   "It would be interesting to trace his illness as it progressed and the way everyone around him reacted to it."

S.N.   "Well, soon after he developed this pressure in his side, things really did disintegrate in the household. They fought all of the time."

S.N.   "Meal times are a disaster, his symptoms are worse then."

S.N.   "It's probably because trying to eat, or even thinking about eating, makes him feel awful."

S.N.   "Praskovya complains about his temper, she says he always had one, for the 20 years that she has known him. She starts to wonder if he has some physical problem."

S.N.   "Is it natural for her to think that she is praiseworthy? She does think so. She admires herself for her self restraint."

S.N.   "He has become disagreeable pretty much all of the time and she thinks:

> Having come to the conclusion that her husband had a dreadful temper and made her life miserable, she began to feel sorry for herself, and the more she pitied herself the more she hated her husband. She began to wish he would die; yet she did not want him to die because then his salary would cease. And this irritated her against him still more. She considered herself dreadfully unhappy just because not even his death could save her, and though she concealed her exasperation, that hidden exasperation of hers increased his irritations also.
>
> *(Tolstoi, 1960, pp. 120, 121)*

S.N.   "What an awful bind they are in, they hate each other, I think. At least they do sense this in one another. The atmosphere in that household must have been dreadful."

S.N.   "They cannot reach out to one another, pretty sad."

S.N.   "It's at this point that Ivan begins his round of doctor's visits trying to find out what is the matter with him."

S.N.   "He thinks that the doctor treats him with the same important air that he treated people in court with, it doesn't seem to him that the doctor even listened to the answers he gave to his questions. It was as though the doctor had already made up his mind."

S.N.   "Here, at this doctor's office, he reminds me of Watanabe because he is trying to find out the truth, 'was his case serious or not?'"

S.N.   "The doctor just goes blithely on, summing up, saying he either has appendicitis or a floating kidney. He talks about Ivan's troubles without any personal regard for him."

S.N.   "Yes, and so what Ivan thinks is that he is in really bad shape, otherwise he would have answered his question directly."

S.N.   "He is stung because he realizes that he has done the very same thing to people in his court."

S.N. "He gets all apologetic, trying to get the doctor to answer his burning question, but the doctor dismisses him without the answer saying;

> I have already told you what I consider necessary and proper. The analysis may show something more.

(Tolstoi, 1960, p. 122)

S.N. "I felt very sorry for Ivan here, he is really sick, he's scared and he gets the run around which only makes him more frightened."

S.N. "But, maybe the doctor didn't know what was wrong with him and couldn't tell him straight out."

S.N. "Maybe, but he could have sympathized with him."

S.N. "Ivan is a proud man who likes to be correct in everything, so it must have been embarrassing for him to beg for an answer like that."

S.N. "The whole downward course of his illness is pretty humiliating, isn't it?"

S.N. "He is very down when he comes home that day, he is sure he has something fatally wrong. This gnawing pain in his side never goes away."

S.N. "Unfortunately, when he gets home he tries to tell Praskovya about the doctor's visit. But Lisa comes in ready to go shopping. Neither the daughter or the wife can sit still long enough to hear what happened."

S.N. "Praskovya says she is happy he went to the doctor, reminds him to take his medicine and she is out the door."

S.N. "I think that it is amazing that what Ivan goes through, personally, is almost exactly what we learned about last year reading Kubler-Ross. The stages of dying were the same in 1886 as they are now."

S.N. "I don't see that in this story at all."

S.N. "It's there, first he is preoccupied with his illness."

S.N. "He monitors all of his symptoms. When things don't happen the way the doctors say they will, he gets more depressed."

S.N. "He also finds other people who are sick and tries to find out all of the details of their illness, or the reason for people's death or recovery. Then he adopts anything that resembles his state."

S.N. "He also tried a kind of mind control, tried forcing himself not to think about what he was experiencing."

S.N. "But that didn't work, anytime he was upset at home or at the office he remembered his illness."

S.N. "Yes, and he would get angry at the person who agitated him, he wasn't angry with himself."

S.N. "Finally, he was on-guard all of the time, just waiting for someone to irritate him."

S.N. "Then he begins making rounds to other specialists."

S.N. "Our patients do the same thing, it's just disguised in the form of second opinions."

S.N. "He also tried homeopathic medicine and a 'wonder working icon.'"

S.N. "Then he drops back to thinking, no, he must stop all of these things and just follow his treatment plan to the letter. If he could do this and not think about being ill he would get better."

S.N. "But we learn that doesn't work:

> The pain in his side oppressed him and seemed to grow worse and more incessant, while the taste in his mouth grew stranger and stranger. It seemed to him that his breath had a disgusting smell, and he was conscious of a loss of appetite and strength. There was no deceiving himself: something terrible, new, and more important than anything before in his life, was taking place within him of which he alone was aware.
>
> *(Tolstoi, 1960, p. 125)*

S.N. "Do you notice what is happening here? Ivan's family went on with their lives as usual, yet they were angry with him for dragging them down. The wife and daughter blame him for being ill."

S.N. "He has been exiled in his own home. Just like Philoktetes was exiled. It's just the same."

S.N. "Horrible to have this in your own home."

S.N. "His colleagues exile him too. Sometimes with sympathetic gestures that remind him he is ill and weak. Mostly, there is an air that he has poisoned the lives of others because of his state."

S.N. "I tried to imagine what he was feeling and I couldn't. I always thought that when a family member got sick, others felt sorry for them and helped care for them."

S.N. "Also, he saw himself wasting away, literally looked into a mirror and saw his thinness."

S.N. "He overheard his brother-in-law tell Praskovya that he was 'a dead man.'"

S.N. "Sick people are very sensitive about their appearance. They don't want to look sick. They don't want people to look at them differently, or treat them differently."

S.N. "Meanwhile, there is this dreadful blackness hanging over him. He thought about it all of the time."

S.N. "I know why, or maybe I should say, one of the reasons why, ill people don't want others to look at them differently . . . it's because it is a loss. I mean, if people don't see you the same as before, that is a loss."

S.N. "Also, it is kind of a vicious circle. You feel sick, you look sick, but you are trying not to think about it all of the time. Then you perceive others looking at you differently, maybe treating you differently; that can only remind you, once again, that you are sick. In other words, nothing will let you forget your illness."

S.N. "So then, it isn't just that Ivan and Philoktetes were exiled by others' lack of care. They were set apart because of their cancer and erupting infection."

S.N. "And then, because of what the illness did to them. You know, for Ivan, the cancer gives him foul breath, gnawing, constant pain, it ruins every meal."

S.N. "He can't even enjoy his friends and bridge games anymore, let alone perform at work. And he quarrels even more with his wife."

S.N. "You notice him looking at himself differently, too. He feels he is disappearing right before his very eyes."

S.N. "One of his biggest losses is self-control. He loses so much strength he cannot even get on and off a commode without help, can't even dress himself. That is a terrible loss."

S.N.   "Philoktetes' foul smelling wound and his constant complaining of pain set him apart from all of his troops."

S.N.   "And the combination of 10 years of exile and constant pain made him very angry and bitter."

S.N.   "I think that both of these men were taken over by their pain. Both of them talked about the pain as 'it,' almost another presence."

S.N.   "You can understand that if you have ever had serious pain, when it is in full force it's all you can think about. You can't read, work or anything. It takes over."

S.N.   "It works on you just like Ivan said."

S.N.   "Hard to understand why that has to happen. And, really, having constant pain sets you apart from others, too."

S.N.   "Being angry all of the time can truly set you apart from others."

S.N.   "I am surprised that, in this discussion, no one has mentioned Gerasim. Though he is called a house servant, he really is Ivan's carer. He is not embarrassed by Ivan's illness. He helps him with all of his personal care."

S.N.   "And he always manages to preserve Ivan's dignity."

S.N.   "As I was saying, he is a large figure in this story because he admits to Ivan that he knows *he is dying and he is the only one that does.*"

S.N.   "Gerasim also helps Ivan greatly by holding up his legs so that his belly and side will be less painful."

S.N.   "It's his straight forward, pleasant manner that cheers Ivan. He is the only person that he can tolerate, even when he isn't having pain."

S.N.   "We should mention the opium that was given to Ivan for pain because when he began questioning his life, the way he had lived, he didn't want to be medicated. He didn't want the fuzzy thinking it caused. So, he refused it towards the end."

S.N.   "I suppose he would feel that he had more control without the opium."

S.N.   "Ultimately, what set Ivan apart from all the others in his life was not just the terrible symptoms of the cancer. It was the lie everyone was living. Not one single family member talked to him."

S.N. "When I think about that I imagine that it is because of their fear and ignorance that they can't approach Ivan. I don't think they were used to talking over serious matters."

S.N. "Fear is the key element in this story from my point of view. Ivan was afraid of what the illness would do to him. All the rest were afraid of what it would do to them, or cost them."

MORTALITY AND THE SOUL

S.N. "It is this part of Ivan's story that taught me the most. I have already seen family members do awful things to one another, but I had never realized what it was like for someone when they were facing certain death. I mean, what they thought about, how they thought, how their mind turned over and over."

S.N. "I agree, it's funny to think of people having these dialogues where they talk to someone, either a lost friend or spouse, or, as it is here, to God. I talk like this sometimes when I'm scared or nervous, but I guess I never thought about others doing it, too."

S.N. "These inner conversations begin when Ivan turns away from the hope that he would get comfort from anyone close to him, or any of his friends."

S.N. "They take off when he starts reviewing his life, certain that it will cheer him. But he learns differently because he cannot find many times in his entire life when he was really connected to another person."

S.N. "Not surprising, he was, as we said, a 'comme il faut' guy."

S.N. "Still he is a very brave man, it takes guts to face past deeds."

S.N. "It is courage, despite the weeping, because he doesn't know where it will lead. He is facing the unknown."

S.N. "He questions God, 'What did I do to deserve this?' Not an uncommon question, all of the pain and suffering feel like punishment."

S.N.   "He is talking with God, he wants answers:

> Why has Thou done all this? Why hast Thou brought
> me here? Why, why dost Thou torment me so terribly?
>
> *(Tolstoi, pp. 146, 147)*

S.N.   "To me his courage is mixed with pleading:

> Go! Strike me! But what is it for? What have I done to
> Thee? What is it for?
>
> *(Tolstoi, p. 147)*

S.N.   "He is desperate to know why he must suffer so, but he doesn't shrink from the pain."

S.N.   "No, but he hears another voice within saying:

> What is it you want?
>
> *(Tolstoi, p. 147)*

S.N.   "He repeats this over and over and then answers:

> What do I want? To live and not to suffer. And again
> he listened with such concentrated attention that even
> his pain did not distract him. 'To live? How?' asked his
> inner voice. Why, to live as I used to—well and pleas-
> antly. As you lived before, well and pleasantly?
>
> *(Tolstoi, 1960, p. 147)*

S.N.   "It is apparent to him now that he has led a shallow life, but his mind can't hang on to that thought. I think that is be-cause he is so grooved into thinking that everything he thought or did was proper, so how could it be shallow?"

S.N.   "He suffers in this way for more than 10 days, can you imagine it?"

S.N.   "And then the big question comes;

> What is this? Can it be that it is Death? And the
> inner voice answered; 'Yes, it is Death.' Why these

sufferings? And the voice answered, 'For no reason—
they just are so.'

(Tolstoi, p. 149)

S.N. "This is the most heart breaking part—when he thinks that
maybe his whole life has been wrong. The emotion that he
must have been feeling then most surely was guilt."

S.N. "No, remorse is more like it, he thinks;

> But if that is so, he said to himself, and I am leaving
> this life with the consciousness that I have lost all that
> was given me and it is impossible to rectify it—what
> then?

(Tolstoi, p. 152)

S.N. "Now his remorse and sorrow are at their worst, he looks at
his family and thinks their life together was all a huge deception—a deception which hid both life and death from
them—and him."

S.N. "The details of his death are so real, it made me wonder if
Tolstoi had a near death experience. I mean, falling through
a black sack, feeling pushed by some force."

S.N. "And with all of his will, he struggles against the force. But,
then, the force strikes him in the chest and he has trouble
breathing."

S.N. "And then he is falling through a hole and he sees great light.
It does seem like Tolstoi knew a great deal about dying."

S.N. "It may be that there was a physical force, such as a hemorrhage or something. I don't deny that, of course. But, to me,
what allowed him to let go and die was something else. That
something was his actually forgiving himself for not having
lived a more honest life."

S.N. "I agree, and this happens because, as he is struggling, his
hand touches his son's head and the boy catches it and presses
it to his lips and begins to cry."

S.N. "At that moment, Ivan knew that not only his son was weeping, but also his wife. And he feels sorry for them for the first
time since he became ill. Maybe even longer ago than that."

S.N.   "And he thinks to himself that he must release them and himself from these sufferings. From that moment on he no longer has pain."

S.N.   "This is a vivid picture of the reasons why moral suffering intensifies physical pain."

S.N.   "And moral suffering seems to intensify fear. I don't think it's just that a person expects punishment. It's more that when, for instance, Ivan is struggling with the reality that he led a shallow life, he feared death. He had no hope. All there was was the void, 'the abyss.'"

S.N.   "When he was living that shallow life, he and all the people around him acted as though there was no such thing as death."

S.N.   "We began by talking about the way his colleagues and wife reacted to his death at his funeral. In a way we have come full circle because these individuals are displaying all of the behaviors that Ivan faced at his death. We don't know what they did at their deaths. But they never knew what Ivan faced."

S.N.   "I am not convinced that it would be possible for them to face their deaths the same way that Ivan did."

S.N.   "But you don't know. Just as we don't know what our patients think about either."

S.N.   "But, we know of this possibility, what Ivan faced, how it affected him. We haven't talked about the soul or the human spirit specifically. But, if you think of the soul being made up of the elements that the priest wrote about at the time of the Burghers incident, then you can imagine that it is the whole inner person."

S.N.   "Refresh my memory."

S.N.   "This English priest said the faculties of the soul were the three major ones of Mind (which includes Memory), Reason, and Will, and two minor ones, Imagination and Sensuality.'" (Anonymous, 1961)

S.N.   "Thinking about Ivan this way gives me a real sense of the huge struggle that Ivan waged."

S.N.   "Why?"

S.N.   "Well, the way I see it, he was a victim of the way he thought about living a life. So, in his memory, he reviews his doing things the way people in authority over him expected. It affected the way he perceived absolutely everything in his life. It effected his decisions, judgment, socializing, everything."

S.N. "I think I see where you are going with this. The faculties of his soul, the way he thinks, what he remembers, how he exercises his will are centered on one single premise, 'comme il faut.'"

S.N. "Right. And so it isn't surprising that he has little imagination or isn't spontaneously loving."

S.N. "Then it is some kind of miracle that he was able to go against this force at the end of his life."

S.N. "Yes, his character, his nature wasn't actually open to what it means to pay attention to one's spiritual life."

S.N. "Well, then, this is a hopeful story. In the end, Ivan had hope for himself."

S.N. "This gives you hope that you can look at your own spirit, your own inner life."

S.N. "Yes, but it is also scary. What if we are grooved into similar ways of thinking? What if our judgment is clouded by some way we think, that we don't even know about?"

S.N. "We might as well face it, the big question that Ivan asked that started him on this roller coaster exploration, we will have to face one day. And, in one way or another, most of the people that we care for face, too. I think it is 'the question':

> When I am not, what will there be? There will be nothing. Then where shall I be when I am not anymore: Can this be dying? No, I don't want to!
>
> *(Tolstoi, p. 130)"*

S.N. "Fear would not be a strong enough word to describe what I feel when I think about this. It's bad enough when I think of my mother and father dying, or my brothers or sister. It is the abyss."

S.N. "My mind can't even stay on the subject. It makes me feel very anxious to think I wouldn't have them with me any more. Would they live on somehow?"

S.N. "What would you say to a patient who asked you about life after death?"

S.N.   "I think I would ask them what they thought."

S.N.   "Easy out, they might ask you if you believed in it or not."

S.N.   "That is a very personal question."

S.N.   "I know, but we might be asked, and I would like to be prepared."

S.N.   "Well, it depends on what you were taught when you were a kid. I, for instance, think that there is an after-life. We are in a different form, but it is our spirit."

S.N.   "I don't think there is life after death. We live on in the memory of others."

S.N.   "Isn't hope the central thing here?"

S.N.   "Maybe it is somehow, because when Ivan asked the question he was really terrorized, he was in despair. But when, in the end, he forgave himself and his family, he felt hope."

S.N.   "I don't understand that hope, not really."

S.N.   "To me, the forgiveness released him from the anger and despair. It's as though he was filled with anger and despair, but when he had the desire to forgive, the desire somehow sprung him loose from this anger and despair. And then he felt hopeful."

S.N.   "It's true, if you are despairing, you feel all is lost, so hope is not a possibility. And then, if all is lost, nothing makes any difference."

S.N.   "But wait, what made a difference here was the genuine sadness he saw in his son. He felt it and he responded to it, he realized he loved his son. I mean, he felt this love, whereas, before he just performed like a father."

S.N.   "I think that this love he suddenly felt made him, at last, sensitive to other's suffering."

S.N.   "It also made him appreciate his own somehow."

S.N.   "A funny thing to think about, but I think you are right. Somehow, before this Ivan suffered, even asked 'Why me?' and other questions. But, at the end, I don't know, but somehow it is as though he knew that what he suffered was important, or worthwhile or something."

CONCLUSION

There is an inherent desire to not only understand but also to overcome the pain and mystery of loss. It is, perhaps, the most urgent and least appreciated theme underlying many of the perplexing interactions that students encounter. Here, students grapple with this eternal question, trying to come to terms with what happened to this ordinary man, Ivan Ilych, in his last illness. It is because of Ivan's ordinariness that his life seems so threatening and so terrible. The all-encompassing fear that is at the core of fatal illness may exile family from the dying, and the dying from family, and from him or herself. Those who provide care and assistance to the fatally ill are forced to face the implications of mortality for others and themselves. The moral and spiritual suffering of Ivan in the exile of his illness eventually leads to forgiveness and hope. These students have discovered that in Ivan's spiritual exile, his state of soul became his only concern.

The following pen sketches presented in the "Faces of Loneliness" were written by a student in response to the desolate states of soul she witnessed as a home health aide and as a student nurse. They correspond to the states of exile of illness and old age experienced by Ivan Ilych.

The Faces of Loneliness
by Jodi Osterhout

LONELINESS: The quality or condition of being lonely.

1. Want of society or company; the condition of being alone or solitary; solitariness, loneliness.

   a. 1586; that huge and sportful assemblie grew to him a tedious loneliness, esteeming no body founde, since Diaphantus was lost. 1645; it is not good for a man to be alone loneliness is the first thing God's eye nam'd not good. 1841; that man of Loneliness and mystery. 1861; the eccentric habits which belong to a state of loneliness. 1874; the loneliness of her (Elizabeth's) position only reflected the loneliness of her nature.

2. Uninhabited or unfrequented condition or character (or place); desolateness.

> 1746–1747; the deep silence added to the gloomy aspect, and both heightened by the loneliness of the place, greatly increased the solemnity of the scene. 1860; the loneliness of the place was very impressive. 1900; the unrelieved loneliness of mid-ocean.

   b. A lonely spot.

> 1819; in the bowers of mossy loneliness.

3. the feeling of being alone; the sense of solitude; dejection arising from want of companionship of society.

> 1814; he grew up from year to year in loneliness of the soul. His loneliness on the death of Sarah may have prompted him to seek a companion of his old age. 1876; my own secret aches and loneliness.

English Oxford Dictionary

As a home health aide and student nurse, I met and helped a variety of individuals, many of whom were elderly. In most instances, I wasn't given a full history of the client; therefore, I had no idea what to expect when entering a home. I encountered a great deal of loneliness among these numerous clients. Herein are some of their stories.

Mr. Brown lived in a large beautiful Victorian home with many antiques scattered throughout the abundant rooms. He was a tall slender man in his mid seventies. He had white thinning hair and his light blue eyes were sightless. He wore a soiled white undershirt and brown polyester pants that hung on his thin frame. On his feet he wore red socks and old tattered tan slippers that looked as though they had been buried for years. Mr. Brown shuffled his way around his large home feeling his way as he went. He had memorized the floor plan of the old home, from doorway to the slightest bump in the rug. Since his wife's death six years earlier, Mr. Brown had lived alone. He still got tears in his eyes when he spoke of her.

Although his health was failing, Mr. Brown's mind was still very much intact. The only company he received were the many workers who would come into his home, quickly fix a meal, clean up a room, or give him his biweekly bath. When I suggested attending activities at the senior center, he replied that he tried that but the men he talked to were "out of their minds."

After his bath, I asked Mr. Brown if he wanted a cup of coffee. A look appeared on his face, a look I had not seen in the whole hour I had been there. He turned directly toward me, his eyebrows elevated, and mouth opened in an expression of astonishment. Yet, he said nothing. Finally, after a time of silence, he replied that although he didn't drink coffee, or even like it . . . he would love a cup.

June 16, 1991

Mrs. Molter was an older woman, around 70, who was diagnosed with multiple sclerosis. She was a rather big woman with silver hair and deep green eyes. Due to her illness, she was bed and wheelchair bound, with little movement of her arms. She had a colostomy and a foley catheter, and required complete care. She had to be helped out of bed in the morning with a hoyer lift, her catheter needed to be irrigated and colostomy care had to be completed, among other things. And, at four in the afternoon, she was put back to bed and these procedures were repeated.

Entering her home, I noticed several family members wandering about the house. Mrs. Molter was lying on her back in bed with her covers pulled up to her chin. Among the scattered equipment lying above the blankets, on her stomach, were a television remote, the bed controller, a shoehorn, and a bowl that contained bits of leftover brown bananas.

Taking care of Mrs. Molter was a challenge for she was very demanding even to where her shoehorn was placed on the night stand. Her expression rarely changed from the perpetual wrinkled brow and downward-turned mouth. Although she rarely made idle conversation, she voiced her needs quite often. "Pull me to the right a little . . ." "No, a little more . . ." "Pull me to the left a little . . ." "That's too much . . ." These things she would utter for the entire hour. Meanwhile . . . her family wandered about the house consumed by their own world.

June 20, 1991

Mrs. Lacey was a plump woman with rosy cheeks and white hair. In her late fifties she had moved to the area so that she could live closer to her brother. She had previously lived with her sister who had died six months earlier. From that fateful day, Mrs. Lacey's health started to fail. She had just been diagnosed with cancer and was living alone. Her closest relative was 30 minutes away.

When I entered Mrs. Lacey's apartment at three in the afternoon, I found her sitting in the corner of a dimly lit room. She was hunched over, holding her head in her hands. She was wearing a nightgown and her feet were bare. From the shaking of her shoulders, I could see she was crying. When I approached her, she turned away from me and sobbed openly.

June 26, 1991

Arriving at his house, I was greeted by Mr. Kirby's wife who directed me to his room. He gave neither one of us a glance when we entered. I found him lying in bed, cigarette in his mouth, reading the newspaper. Coffee was on the night stand.

Mr. Kirby was a middle-aged man who suffered from severe chronic obstructive pulmonary disease. He was a rugged looking man, who had dark brown hair and dark brown eyes. His face was leathery and deeply scarred from previous acne. It appeared as though he hadn't shaved in a week and his hair was laden with grease. He had the odor of an unwashed body, and his breath smelled of a mixture of smoke and old food. His voice was harsh and full of crackles. Due to his extremely productive cough, speaking at length was not possible. From the few words that were spoken by Mr. Kirby, I learned that he did not want me to touch him. He told me to leave and ordered his wife to walk me out. His wife spoke not a word. She gave me a look of disgust and led me out of the room. As I made my way down the hallway, I noticed numerous photographs, presumably of the Kirby's grandchildren. A small picture on the back of the shelf caught my eye. Looking closer, I realized that it was an old wedding photograph of Mr. and Mrs. Kirby. The picture, unlike the others, was covered with dust. Although she saw me looking at the pictures, Mrs. Kirby remained silent and showed me to the door.

June 26, 1991

A young, vivacious woman with big blue eyes and blonde hair, Mrs. Mullin had everything in life. She was married to a man she deeply loved, had two wonderful children and all of the money she would ever need. Some fifteen years later, Mrs. Mullin was diagnosed with multiple sclerosis and shortly thereafter, when her condition suddenly worsened, she and her husband were divorced.

The afternoon assignment was to simply help Mrs. Mullin onto the toilet. Entering her home, I found her sitting in her electric wheelchair with a big smile on her face. Although it was not an unpleasant smile, I could sense its thinness. She was a beautiful woman, around 40, well groomed and dressed in black slacks and a red blouse.

When it was time to begin, she instructed me on how to manipulate the wheelchair, for she had no strength in her hands. As we made our way to the bathroom, Mrs. Mullin spoke about her children, both of whom were in college. One was in Boston, the other in Florida.

Helping Mrs. Mullin onto the toilet was not an easy task. She instructed my every move, from how to take apart the wheelchair, to how to manipulate her legs into a position most favorable to her.

When the 15 minutes allotted were over, I helped Mrs. Mullin back into the chair and gathered my things in order to leave. From outside the house I could still see her sitting as I had found her, smiling that uneasy smile, unable to move until the next home care visit.

June 30, 1991

The smell of urine and smoke penetrated the room. There, sitting amongst a pile of magazines, old food, cigarettes, photographs and various other "stuff," that she termed her "life," sat Mrs. Francelli. From her history, it was assumed that hidden in that pile was also a bottle of gin.

Because of her leathery, wrinkled face, her relative youth seemed lost. She had wavy brown hair and big green eyes. Her body was emaciated from poor nutrition, and her teeth yellowed from coffee and cigarettes. She wore light blue, urine-soaked pants and a pink, coffee stained sweatshirt. Socks were all she would ever wear on her feet.

Mrs. Francelli's life consisted of waking up at eleven o'clock in the morning, struggling to get to the bathroom, and then retiring to her chair for the remainder of the day. Surrounding her chair was everything she needed; her phone, a television remote, Kleenex paper, pens, books and resting nearby, her commode, which she rarely used. She sat in her chair all day, watching television programs geared to the mind of a 12-year-old, awaiting the next meals on wheels to appear. The occasional phone calls she received were usually to confirm home care visits.

Dirty jokes were Mrs. Francelli's specialty. She would talk for hours about her life stories and they always had a humorous component. She rarely talked with you, but rather at you, for her hearing was severely impaired. Across the room or even downstairs one could still hear her gabbing away. Whoever walked into the house was subjected to a story or a joke. From the mailman to the home health aide, Mrs. Francelli was desperate to speak to anyone . . . anyone who would come for a "visit."

June 30, 1991

5

The Exile of Emotional Disorder: Bernanos, *Mouchette*, and Cather, "Paul's Case"

People generally think that suicide is an act like any other, the last link in a chain of reflections, or at least of mental images, the conclusion of a supreme debate between the instinct to live and another, more mysterious instinct of renouncement and refusal. But it is not like that. Apart from certain abnormal exceptions, suicide is an inexplicable and frighteningly sudden event, rather like the kind of rapid chemical decompositions which currently-fashionable science can only explain with absurd or contradictory hypotheses.

Bernanos, 1966, p. 119

CLASS DISCUSSION

Prior to class meetings, students closely read and annotated these two stories. These annotations were guided by several question: How do the lives of these two teenagers compare and contrast with one another? What evidence is there that tells us how Paul and Mouchette

Portions of the précis appeared in *Clinical Nurse Specialist: The Journal for Advanced Nursing Practice.*

MOUCHETTE

Bernanos, Georges. (1937). *Mouchette*. Translated from the French *Nouvelle histoire de Mouchette*. (1966). by J. C. Whitehouse. New York: Holt, Rinehart and Winston.

The Characters

Mouchette, 14 year-old French girl

Mother of Mouchette

Father of Mouchette

Mouchette's brothers

Infant son of Mouchette's parents

Madame, the village school mistress

Arséne, friend of Mouchette's father, a game poacher

Ménétrier, the farmer who is the last person to see Mouchette alive

Monsieur Mathieu, Game Warden

Madame Mathieu, Game Warden's wife

Madame Derain, widow, owner of Baker's Shop

Philomene, the village veilleuse (mourner, preparer of the dead for burial)

Mouchette is an illuminating glance into the mind of a destitute, abused, 14-year-old French girl as she lives the last 24 hours of her life. We are shown how Mouchette subjectively perceives events and relationships with her classmates, family, and community. We learn about the ways in which she attempts to survive their cruelty and

(Continued on page 108.)

perceived their classmates, teachers, families, and community members? How did they perceive themselves? How did they think about their worlds? What are the antecedents of their suicides? And finally, what do we learn about their inner states in the last hours of their lives? Note the depth and variety of the responses as they unfold.

S.N.   "Mouchette's and Paul's stories are very, very upsetting to me."

S.N.   "Two young teenagers taking their own lives, how horrible!"

S.N.   "I know, I thought that people who committed suicide were crazy, or really disturbed. But, I don't think that Mouchette and Paul were psychotic or anything like that."

S.N.   "Teenage suicide is more common than you think. In my high school there were two. At least some said they were both suicides. This guy deliberately drove his car into a tree after he lost his girl friend. He was also very drunk at the time."

S.N.   "Who was the other one?"

S.N.   "A classmate of mine who killed herself her freshman year at college. They found her in her room after she had been missing from classes for several days. She had taken an overdose of something."

S.N.   "Was she terribly upset about something? Is that why she did it?"

S.N.   "She was failing all of her classes, she couldn't study. She didn't have friends there. She was mixed up, oh, I don't know. I'm still very sad about what happened to her."

S.N.   "We learned in another class that teenagers can get very depressed and if they have trouble at home and in school and with friends, they are at great risk."

S.N.   "Also, like this boy just described, if they have difficulties with the boyfriend or girlfriend. And, of course, it is extremely dangerous if they are doing drugs, then everything falls apart for them."

S.N.   "I know of a very studious, shy girl, actually. She was a nervous sort of kid. Well, she missed out on some scholastic award she tried for. She tried to take her life, too. She had always gotten all A's and I think she was not only disappointed but also embarrassed that she didn't win."

mockery as she struggles with her own confused thoughts about becoming a woman. Her astute observations and obstinacy have assured her safety until she is befriended and deceived by a friend of her father's who brutally rapes her. In the aftermath, she struggles vainly to regain her only possession, her pride.

Sensitized by events in the story, we come to admire Mouchette's tenacity and to appreciate more vividly the stigma that enshrouds destitution. Crucial to our understanding of Mouchette's character is the fact that she is more perceptive of people's motives than are her affluent classmates and school mistress. Her ways of knowing come from a sure recognition of others' true intentions as revealed by a tone of voice, a gesture, or a glance. She is acutely aware of her own effect upon others in just this same way. She studies people's hands and comes to the realization that "hands do not lie": they, in fact, tell a person's story. She knows her own rough, thick hands expose her difficult life and heritage.

Following the deception and betrayal of Arséne, her father's friend, she blames herself for the brutal rape. And she yearns for comfort and understanding from other women in the village in the absence of her deceased mother. A baker's wife, whom she had helped in the past, is affected by Mouchette's dismay, but once she discovers the reason for it, cruelly repels her, calling her a slut. Another, younger woman whom Mouchette physically reaches out to for solace presses mercilessly for details of the rape. Mouchette detects the repulsion the woman holds for her and she desperately flees this woman, sensing that to share her dismay and her secret would only add to her shame. Bernanos reminds us that this facile kind of pity which insists on the relating of sordid details is not true compassion. This woman even offers to pay Mouchette if she will come back the next day to tell her more of what happened.

A third woman, the designated village mourner, who has, in her old age, come to perversely enjoy death, waylays Mouchette by

(Continued on page 110.)

S.N.   "How can you all talk so freely about this? You don't know what was on these teenagers' minds. Maybe there was lots more that nobody will ever know."

S.N.   "If these kids were anything like Paul and Mouchette, then there is plenty more to know."

S.N.   "True, for one thing, these two were loners, they had no one to pal around with, nobody their age to hang out with."

S.N.   "Also, they never got any guidance or advice from their parents."

S.N.   "In fact, Paul's mother died when he was a baby and Mouchette's mother died during the story, so to speak."

S.N.   "We should say, then, that the loss of a parent figures in somehow."

S.N.   "Of course this makes a difference, but it also makes a difference if you have been close to the parent, or never known them. It is a very private, individual matter."

S.N.   "Well, neither one of these two teenagers ever knew the tenderness and care of a mother, for what that's worth. Paul never knew his, and Mouchette's was so subject to her alcoholic husband and sick baby, and then her own illness, that she wasn't available to Mouchette."

S.N.   "I want to talk about the teachers in both of these stories because I think that they were appalling!"

S.N.   "Their teachers thoroughly disliked them. They openly ridiculed them in front of their classmates."

S.N.   "In a way, what happens to Paul is the real shocker because the principal and all of the teachers are going after him together! They don't check one another. It's like, I don't know, the opening scene is like a lynching. I am amazed he gets to re-enter school."

S.N.   "Neither Paul or Mouchette had one single advocate, not one."

S.N.   "In both of these stories, the teenagers are totally adrift, they are not connected to anyone at all."

S.N.   "It isn't uncommon for 14-year-olds to feel that they are not connected to anyone. Nor to realize that they hate their families. That would be the normal teenager. Also, many kids that age have trouble relating to their community."

S.N.   "We are talking about something much more serious here. Sure, the public in general doesn't especially like teenagers, they are so all over the place."

weaving a strange, spellbinding story of a young girl's death. The old woman romanticizes the child's death saying she willfully gave up her life for that of another. She even gives Mouchette a dress which once belonged to the dead girl. Then she cleverly extracts the degrading details of the rape from Mouchette, leaving her humiliated once again.

The failure of these village women to sincerely help Mouchette is worthy of our closest scrutiny. They are especially culpable. They all knew that she had just lost her mother, they see her obvious physical and mental distress, and they strangely relish the fact that she has been brutalized and raped. One judges and condemns the vulnerable 14-year-old for her poverty and for the dastardly behavior of a man. Another indulges her perverse fascination with sordid accounts of other people's sufferings. Most dreadful of all is the old woman who plants the idea of death as a seductive alternative to life, knowing full well that Mouchette is a vulnerable, ignorant, wounded child. Mouchette, in her innocence, cannot find a solution to her unbearable condition of life. Stripped of her dignity and shamed by violence and the willful, self-serving, supposedly respected women of the village, she succumbs to the impulse to suicide.

S.N.   "There are plenty of articles that talk about the teen years as some kind of psychosis."

S.N.   "My parents had a book—something like *Understanding Your Teen*—that helped them deal with my brothers and myself. I used to hear them talking about us to their friends."

S.N.   "But the disorder that Paul and Mouchette found themselves in was far more serious than typical teen stuff."

S.N.   "I know, and I have been thinking about them in relation to others that we have talked about in this course."

S.N.   "Me, too. And I think that they both had a lot of courage, they went bravely on every day knowing that everyone was mocking them in one way or another."

S.N.   "Perhaps with the exception of Paul when he was ushering at Carnegie Hall for the classical music concerts."

S.N.   "True, people that he ushered to seats there thought he was charming and responsible."

S.N.   "I am trying to remember if Mouchette ever enjoyed even one minute of such a feeling of admiration."

S.N.   "I think that she did, the night before she died. It happened with Arséne and maybe that is what affected her the most. I mean, what influenced her opinions of him. He complimented her on her bravery for not crying when her father beat her in public. And then, he told her he had always liked her."

S.N.   "There is another thing. And I think that this is especially important. Here she is, always alone, defiant, suspicious of everyone. And then, when Arséne falls ill with the epileptic seizure, she feels a tenderness towards him. She had never felt tenderness for another person in her life before this."

S.N.   "I personally think that both of these children felt superior in a very particular way."

S.N.   "That really surprises me, I don't see that at all."

S.N.   "Well, Paul's fantasies of the glorious life of the rich in New York plus the opportunity to be among theatre people lifted him out of his anxious state. And I think that because he had these fantasies, and he knew others didn't, he felt a kind of superiority."

S.N.   "I disagree, it is more likely that he felt inferior all of the time and that caused him to have the fantasies."

"PAUL'S CASE"

Cather, Willa. (1989). "Paul's Case" in *Great Short Stories of Willa Cather*. New York: Harper and Row.

Characters in the Story

Paul, 14 year-old teenage boy attending Pittsburgh High School

Teachers at Pittsburgh High School

Principal of High School

Charley Edwards, actor friend of Paul's

Paul's father

Paul's sisters

Taxi drivers in New York & Newark

In "Paul's Case," we meet Paul, a young teenage boy as he appears before his high school teachers petitioning for his school suspension to be lifted. The vehemence of their disdain and merciless attack on him is surprising since his "misdemeanors" don't seem particularly serious. His apparent dislike of his teachers, and flamboyant, theatrical way of dressing, don't seem to be enough to warrant the torment they are putting him through, though his lying and incomplete school work are flagrant transgressions. Paul, himself, sees nothing wrong with the lies he tells. To him they are "indispensable for overcoming friction" (Cather, 1989, p. 64). He is allowed to re-enter school and as the last weeks of his life unfold, an indelible tale is imprinted upon us.

Paul, we see, has been misread and misunderstood by all those around him. They have interpreted his fragility as purposeful flamboyance, his lying as insolence, his smart, clever remarks as deliberate

(Continued on page 114.)

S.N.   "It seems to me that he hated, or should I say, disliked, being with most of the people he knew in his family and at school. He felt repelled by them. The fantasies were his retreat, the way he tolerated life."

S.N.   "And the fantasies were imaginings of a better life, not weird things. He pictured himself in other surroundings, he couldn't stand his own. He used to get sick when he had to come home to Cordelia Street."

S.N.   "Mouchette felt a kind of superiority because she taunted her classmates and people in the village. She purposely provoked doing things like rolling in the mud in front of people just coming out of Mass."

S.N.   "The way that they dressed set them apart from others, too. Of course, Mouchette had no choice, really. Her family was desperately poor. But Paul chose to dress very strangely. He would wear ascots, flowers in his lapels. You could say he dressed theatrically just to go to school."

S.N.   "It doesn't take much imagination to picture what the other kids made of that!"

S.N.   "Both of them were skillful liars, too. But their lying had different elements, they didn't do it for the same reasons. Paul did it to avoid friction. He knew it was wrong but didn't see the harm in trying to avoid confrontations. Mouchette didn't really think it was wrong. Bernanos said that '. . . lying had never seemed wrong to Mouchette, for it was the most precious—probably ˙the only—privilege of the wretched.'" (Bernanos, 1966, p. 67)

S.N.   "That tells me that she lied simply to survive, she knew she had to, and she was not ashamed of it."

S.N.   "Both Paul and Mouchette were very perceptive. They could tell a person's motives by the tone of voice, the look in the eye. Mouchette had this way of watching people's hands as they talked. She could tell whether they were being honest or not by what their hands were doing as they talked."

S.N.   "But, neither of them had any counsel from an adult. As far as I'm concerned, their teachers were nearly hopeless. These two teenagers must have been just about the neediest kids in their classes and they abused them terribly instead of helping them."

taunts. Save for one, his drawing teacher, they have united into an unthinking, undiscerning pack which has turned upon this physically and emotionally delicate boy whose main pastime is fantasizing. He simply cannot bear the monotony and mediocrity of his lower-middle-class life. Instead, he lives for his associations with the world of the arts and the theatre. Only fine music and the smells of the theatre can energize him. He is enchanted by performers and their appearance of fame and fortune.

His reactions to events and to those around him affect his every mood. He cannot bear close association with any member of his family. The only boy with older sisters, he lost his mother in infancy. His father, an uneducated small business man, opposes all Paul cares about. When his exasperated father pulls him out of school and secures a full time job for him, severing his ties with the world of the arts, Paul is devastated.

As with Mouchette, Paul cannot convey his inner state to anyone. He, too, can sense other people's motives and the way in which they are repelled by him, but his temperament is vastly different from hers. He only feels that life is worth living when he imagines himself in a world of glitter and celebrity. And while this does not seem attainable, his sense of dread at facing an existence away from that world leads him to steal funds from the company and flee to New York. There, for one glorious week, he lives the life he feels is meant for him, buying expensive clothes, eating the best food, attending the Opera. As the week closes in on him and he reads of his theft in the newspapers, he knows that his father will find him and take him home to the life he cannot bear.

Paul cannot think of a solution to his dilemma and those around him find no solution either. Unable to imagine any other life than the one in New York, he flees the hotel before his father arrives. In his last moments of life, when death is inevitable, he realizes other possibilities. Sadly, no one ever knew that his inner life consisted only of fantasies by which he measured his and others' worth.

S.N.   "Kids this age need counsel from adults, even if they don't want it. They don't know how to think through things that upset them. They don't know how to make decisions. They have trouble tolerating intense emotions."

S.N.   "It's almost as though Mouchette and Paul were foreigners in their own home towns. They didn't communicate with others and the others around them thought they were strange, undesirable, so they either ignored them or even mocked them. Foreigners are sometimes treated this way."

S.N.   "It is almost as though they don't speak the same language, isn't it?"

S.N.   "For Paul, it was more that his interests were so different from his classmates and his teachers."

S.N.   "And for Mouchette, it was almost as though she couldn't speak, she rarely had conversations with anyone."

S.N.   "They did notice the way others dressed and behaved. Mouchette used to hide in the bushes after school to spy on the other girls, to listen to what they talked about."

S.N.   "She was just beginning to be interested in boys. But, Paul didn't notice his classmates much at all, boys or girls."

S.N.   "He was more absorbed in the detailed fantasies he had created."

S.N.   "I don't imagine that either one of them learned very much in school."

S.N.   "Probably not, they both missed a great deal of school."

S.N.   "We could go on and on looking for all of the reasons why Paul and Mouchette were exiles in their own communities and homes, but it seems to me that, painful as it will be, we should look very closely at what happened to them in their final hours that led them to suicide."

S.N.   "Then I would go back to the beginning of Mouchette's story when we learn that though she is aware of the misery that her father's alcoholism inflicts she never dwelt on what happened during the episodes when he came home drunk and angry. Bernanos tells how her mind worked, especially when reflecting on the circumstances of her life.

> ... thoughts never passed through Mouchette's mind
> in such a logical way. She was vague and jumped

> quickly from one thing to another. If the very poor could associate the various images of their poverty they would be overwhelmed by it, but their wretchedness seems to them to consist simply of an endless succession of miseries, a series of unfortunate chances.

(Bernanos, 1966, p. 16)

S.N. "That partially explains why she reacted as she did towards her hateful teacher. This teacher purposely humiliated Mouchette many, many times before her classmates. She would insist she sing when she didn't want to, she provoked her, too. But, surprisingly, Mouchette didn't hate her. She didn't really hate anyone.

> She was not aware of despising anyone because, in her innocence, this seemed outside her capabilities and she thought no more of it than she did of the other more material characteristics which the rich and powerful reserve for themselves.

(Bernanos, 1966, pp. 30, 31)

S.N. "It's as though she doesn't imagine that she has certain human rights. I mean, if a person is mistreated, they should be able to react to it. I think that she did, but she somehow didn't store up incidences, she didn't keep score."

S.N. "It is hard for me to imagine someone's life so filled with miseries that the actual events no longer register. Or they somehow don't hold the weight of what has happened."

S.N. "She did see herself as a rebel though, '. . . a rebel against an order which the school mistress typified.' (Bernanos, 1966, p. 31) She wasn't ashamed of being told she was no good, and she wasn't ashamed of the rags she dressed in."

S.N. "Somehow, though, and I don't exactly understand why, she was ashamed of her singing voice. And Bernanos says it is a beautiful, fragile voice, far superior to the voices of her classmates."

S.N. "I know, and when she refuses to sing, the teacher somehow feels deprived."

S.N.   "I think that it's possible that she felt vulnerable when she sang in front of her classmates, and she doesn't want to feel that way. She has this persona of the rebel."

S.N.   "Have you thought that her voice unnerves her when she hears it? Because it was, in a way, unlike her to possess such a voice. You know that it was special because her classmates envy her."

S.N.   "She wouldn't be aware of why it upsets her, she doesn't reflect on things day to day."

S.N.   "Thinking things over for her is an enormous effort. The way her mind worked was to react at the moment, but always to survive. She wouldn't have tried to understand what occurred in the classroom."

S.N.   "When Mouchette was younger she was similar to Paul. She used to day dream. But by the time we meet her she no longer could even day dream.

> By dreaming she often managed to escape from herself, but it was a long time since she had lost the secret of those mysterious ways by which one entered into oneself.
>
> *(Bernanos, 1966, p. 33)*

S.N.   "The night after school that she gets lost in the storm is typical of any other day. Mouchette left school early, hid in the bushes to spy on the other girls and then started off through the woods toward home."

S.N.   "But losing her way in the woods is her undoing, the beginning of the end because this is when Arséne finds her. And by the time he does she is nearly exhausted. When I think of all of the things that we know about her and imagine her in the dark, alone, it freaks me out. She was truly vulnerable and Arséne knew it."

S.N.   "By the time that Arséne rescues her and takes her to the hunter's cabin, she is not thinking the way she usually does, she is very concentrated. She senses things happening to her in a far different way than ever before."

S.N.   "At first, though, I think that she was taken in by Arséne's tale of a dangerous cyclone-like storm brewing."

S.N.   "Also, she knows he is a poacher who has had trouble with the law before, her father knows a lot of such persons. So, when Arséne tells her that he had a fight with the Game Warden and accidently killed him, she believes it."

S.N.   "So, really, in a very few minutes he has Mouchette afraid to go outside because of this storm. And then, he has made her an accomplice, in a way, to this murderous deed."

S.N.   "But, there are other things that occur that create a powerful emotional upheaval in Mouchette. She has a physical reaction to him. I mean that he awakens in her emotions that are completely new to her. And, I think that comes about because he treats her like an adult. She looks at him differently than she has before. She had seen him any number of times with her father."

S.N.   "He is different, too, this time he has something on his mind in regard to her."

S.N.   "I don't think that he rescued her with rape on his mind. But it evolved to that . . . events led up to that."

S.N.   "I don't believe that, why else lie about the storm, and lie about the murder? The Game Warden was alive and well."

S.N.   "I think that he is conniving. He tells her that he has always admired her, always liked her. And because of this she looks at him differently."

S.N.   "But the event that really affects her is when he cauterizes his wound with a glowing ember from the fire."

S.N.   "This, she thinks, is incredibly brave, and not something she has ever witnessed before. Also, he has an epileptic seizure then because of the intense pain. She has never witnessed a seizure before. She thinks he may have died."

S.N.   "This creates great inner turmoil for her."

S.N.   "But, you know, she has very tender feelings for him, and these tender feelings are very real . . . they are also brand new. She has never felt tender toward another human being before."

S.N.   "I know, all of a sudden, this guy seems dear to her. Startling!"

S.N.   "She tries to take care of him when he loses consciousness and all of a sudden she is singing, and she is not embarrassed."

S.N.   "If only things had ended there, but they don't. After drinking more bad wine, he brutally rapes her. What a coward!"

S.N. "She manages to get free of him and hides in the wood until dawn. You would think that she would detest him. But she doesn't; instead, she feels a terrible shame."

S.N. "It is at this moment that, to me, her life hangs in the balance—she has no one to turn to, she is engulfed in self-blame. And it bothers me no end that she feels ashamed! What about him, he's an absolute cad."

S.N. "The saddest thing is that this happened to her just as she is feeling affection for another person for the first time.

> The violence which had been done to her had taken her at the height of her humble love. She could not feel hatred.
>
> *(Bernanos, 1966, p. 64)*

S.N. "She tries, in her wounded state to gain sympathy from her mother. But the mother is too ill to give it. Mouchette is alone."

S.N. "The village women that she turns to do not help her either. In fact, their behavior boxes her in, isolates her even more. This is a new thing for her, seeking comfort, and they fail her."

S.N. "It is hard to know which of the women is more irresponsible. Mathieu's wife wants to hear all of the details of the rape. This causes Mouchette to experience the shame all over again . . . somehow it is worse to have to tell the story to her."

S.N. "Also, Mouchette is loyal to the core, she doesn't want Arséne arrested for poaching, she intends to keep his secret. She knows she will never see him again, he will run away."

S.N. "The widow who owns the Baker's Shop is brutal, I think. She takes her in, offering solace, then detects evidence of the rape and is caustic with Mouchette. Mouchette can only run away."

S.N. "All this while Mouchette's emotions have not abated, how could they? Instead, they are building. Bernanos says that:

> Once again her fear and her anger turned inwards upon herself; it was herself she hated. Why? What had she done? If only she had done something! No remorse could have caused her more anguish than the

blind incomprehensible shame she carried in her flesh
and blood. As she walked along her fingers clenched
on her breast and pulled at it almost murderously.

(Bernanos, 1966, p. 89)

S.N.   "When Philomene, the village mourner, sees her in such
        distress, she asks her in. But, sadly, she can talk of nothing
        but death. And she romanticized it, too. She mesmerizes
        Mouchette with her tales of the dying, especially one story
        in particular which involves a young girl from her past."

S.N.   "Somehow, without prying, she gets Mouchette to tell her
        what happened."

S.N.   "I know, and somehow Philomene's words allow Mouchette
        to feel sorry for herself."

S.N.   "The thought that lingers is the fact that this young girl
        from the village mourner's past supposedly let go of her life,
        according to the woman, so that she, who was sickly, could
        live."

S.N.   "You can see Mouchette thinking that somehow this was a
        solution, she could remain loyal to Arséne, even though he
        brutalized her."

S.N.   "Another thing to consider is that she has been influenced by
        the magazines with stories of romance and the stars. She
        began at this moment to imagine that her life was to be like
        those, she would be

> Amongst those rare people who provide a tender spec-
> tacle for sensitive souls.
>
> *(Bernanos, 1966, p. 117)*

S.N.   "Though in these last few hours before her death she is very
        confused, with effort she reasoned that she had to make the
        loss of her lover into something wonderful:

> . . . and that all at once she had stepped into the strange
> world that she had sometimes glimpsed in books.
>
> *(Bernanos, 1966, p. 117)*

S.N. "She, somehow, finds herself in the old quarry, a place she has used as a kind of retreat for years."

S.N. "All she can think of at this point is what the old woman said . . . death. And now Mouchette is preoccupied with it. Before this she had vague fear of it, but now she began thinking of her own death,

> with her heart gripped with excitement of a great discovery, the feeling that she was about to learn what she had been unable to learn from her brief experience of love.
>
> *(Bernanos, 1966, p. 118)*

S.N. "But at the same time she is very afraid of death, but she has lost her will, her fight. She experienced the same kind of drowsiness and feeling of disorder that Paul did just before he died."

S.N. "She didn't want to die."

S.N. "Her last hope was Ménétrier who just glanced at her and rode on."

S.N. "She wanted to call out to him but he disappeared like a ghost. He never questioned what she was doing there."

S.N. "Awful, don't you think? There she was, alone, disheveled, sitting on the edge of the water, distraught with the dead girl's dress in her hands. How could he have just gone on his way?"

S.N. "When I read about the last moments of her life, it all seems like a slow moving dark, dark dream. It's as though she is being sucked down into the quarry pool."

S.N. "That is despair overcoming her. She cannot hang onto the wish for revenge, she simply won't betray Arséne. Her old optimism which was so linked to being a rebel is gone. And she has no hope."

S.N. "In the end, though she really, truly didn't want to die, her will dissolved."

DISCUSSION, WEEK #TWO

S.N.   "It's a good thing that the discussions about Paul and Mouchette were separated by a week. Their stories are so sad. I had to force myself to read to the end of both stories. I was afraid of how I would feel about their suicides. They became very real people to me."

S.N.   "I know, I resisted these stories but we will most certainly meet teenagers and adults who were overwhelmed like they were. So, I decided, better that we have a chance to talk about these things before we have to face them in real life."

S.N.   "Paul is a very different kid, very different from Mouchette. He's an American teenager. He comes from a middle-class family who owns a house on a street in Pittsburgh which has families of business men."

S.N.   "Mouchette was a girl from a little French village who lived in poverty. She attended a small village school, whereas Paul attended Pittsburgh High School."

S.N.   "Also, their fantasy lives were vastly different. Mouchette daydreamed as a little girl. But Paul's fantasy life was all consuming. And often times he sought out what triggered it. His after-school job involved it; he was an usher at Carnegie Hall. It is almost as though he was obsessed with this inner life."

S.N.   "What was it that you think triggered his inner world of fantasy?"

S.N.   "It's music, any kind of music. But it is such a trip for him. Cather says that music was all he needed:

> . . . music; any sort of music, from an orchestra to a barrel organ. He needed only the spark, the indescribable thrill that made his imagination master of his senses, and he could make plots and pictures enough of his own.
>
> *(Cather, 1989, p. 77)*

S.N.   "Well, those are not psychotic fantasies at all. Music means a great deal to many, many people. They listen to it to lift their spirits because they simply enjoy it. Some are just addicted to it. You can see it even with all of us. We have our Walkmans, tape decks in our cars. You know how it goes."

S.N.   "I think that one of the differences here with Paul is that the music triggered his fantasy life . . . and the fantasy life was more pleasing and real to him than any aspect of the life he was living. Any aspect that it, except when he was working or with his actor friend."

S.N.   "Lots of people day dream—most people, in fact."

S.N.   "And, also, he knew the difference between reality and his fantasies."

S.N.   "But, the day dreaming affected his school work almost completely. Because he didn't do his school work and had this cavalier attitude about it, he got suspended more than once."

S.N.   "I agree, his after-school associations with the actors of the local theatre made ordinary school life impossible for him. He simply couldn't tolerate the people or places in his life:

> After a night behind the scenes, Paul found the school-room more than ever repulsive; the bare floors and naked wall; the prosy men who never wore frock coats, or violets in their buttonholes; the women with their dull gowns, shrill voices, and pitiful seriousness about prepositions that govern the dative. He could not bear to have the other pupils think, for a moment, that he took these people seriously; he must convey to them that he considered it all trivial, and was there only by way of a jest, anyway.
>
> *(Cather, p. 77)*

S.N.   "He used to tell whoppers, too. He'd say he was having dinner with the actors, or going abroad with them, when he didn't, he'd invent a cover-up story."

S.N.   "This dual life Paul was living went on until one day he told his teachers that he couldn't be bothered with school work any longer, he had to help his actor friends."

S.N.   "To me there is a key event that leads to the death of both of these teenagers. For Mouchette, it was the loss of her dignity. And for Paul, it was the loss of his greatest pleasures. When the principal told his father what he said about helping the actor friends, they agreed that the best thing for Paul would be to take away his involvement with music and the theatre."

S.N.   "It is evident that they really do not understand him because those two things were all he lived for, it was ordinary life that he found ugly."

S.N.   "Right, I see what his father did as the turning point in Paul's story. He gets Paul a job in an ordinary business and forbids him to see the actors again."

S.N.   "Most serious here is that he also talks to Charley Edwards, Paul's *only* friend, insisting that Charley stay away from him. Charley was Paul's favorite, they spent Sunday evenings together because Paul assisted him in dress rehearsals."

S.N.   "But, if I had been his parent, I might have done the same things. He wasn't doing his school work, he was refusing to do it."

S.N.   "He was also staying out all hours of the night with these things that he was doing."

S.N.   "But there must have been some other way to manage the situation."

S.N.   "I don't think that Paul's father knew how fragile he was."

S.N.   "The principal and the teachers, save one, didn't either. And the art teacher, who saw that Paul was fragile, didn't follow through with his concern for him."

S.N.   "Paul's sisters didn't realize his state, either."

S.N.   "Well, I think he had a hell of a lot of courage to do what he did . . . to steal money from the firm and head off for New York City."

S.N.   "And he had it planned out so well, too. He was very clever in getting away with it."

S.N.   "The reason it seems so brave to me is because Paul did it when he lost hope. He knew he couldn't go on in the job his father got for him. It must have taken a great deal of energy, too."

S.N.   "This notion of being in New York was a kind of optimistic endeavor more than hope, I think. Something like what kept Mouchette going. She was a kind of rebel who always looked forward to revenge. She became desolate when she lost her will for revenge."

S.N.   "Right! And Paul became desolate when he lost his will, or should I say desire, for his treasured fantasy life."

S.N.   "In a way he lived through his ideal fantasy. He got himself outfitted with fine clothes and luggage, signed himself into a fancy hotel suite. He was acting the part of someone's rich kid . . . it read just like a novel."

S.N.   "This part of the story was like a movie to me, I could actually picture him eating those fancy dinners."

S.N.   "But as the glorious week spins on you get the sense that things are very time limited, that it is only a matter of days before he is discovered."

S.N.   "But, to go back to his loss of desire, it happened when he read in the newspapers of his crime and, also, that his father was on his way to New York to retrieve him. He realized, with a final certainty, that there was no whopper big enough that he could invent that would cover up the public announcement of what he had done."

S.N.   "It's too bad that his imagination failed him at that point. If it hadn't, he might have imagined that he would be some sort of celebrity amongst the other kids back in Pittsburgh."

S.N.   "He has one more big night in the city, drinks too much and gets ill. He has his plan of what he will do."

S.N.   "I try to imagine his state of mind in those last hours, but I can't."

S.N.   "I think that he was in a state of feeling intensely empty, empty of his optimism and empty of desire. He was convinced that there was only one thing left to do."

S.N.   "That emotional state must feel dreadful . . . a dreadful nothingness is the only way I can think of it."

S.N.   "Cather says that it is only in his last moments that he realized his 'folly,' that what he had decided to do was not his only choice.

>   As he fell, the folly of his haste occurred to him with
>   merciless clearness, the vastness of what he had left un-
>   done. There flashed through his brain, clearer than
>   ever before, the blue of Adriatic water, the yellow of
>   Algerian sands.

(Cather, p. 90)

S.N.   "Neither he nor Mouchette had developed inner resources to cope with important losses. When they lost what they cared about the most in this world, they couldn't figure out how to go on, they couldn't figure out anything to do, nor anyone to turn to. The few people that they saw in the last hours and moments of their lives turned away in indifference."

S.N.   "But worse than that, which is terrible enough, and in itself an exile, is the disorder that they experienced psychologically."

S.N.   "Why do you say that?"

S.N.   "They had both experienced disappointment, of course, but they had not ever felt completely desolate before. And they were unable to cope with it, with the intense emotional state. Revenge and fantasy were no longer possible."

S.N.   "To me it's like an alienation from the self. I don't like that word. Exile is more appropriate somehow. Remember what the English priest said the faculties of the soul were: memory, reason and will. Well, Paul and Mouchette had lost their old ways of reasoning and their will. They were exiled from what they knew themselves to be. The emotionally disordered state led to this."

S.N.   "There is another factor, too. They both were physically and emotionally exhausted. They were so exhausted that they became kind of disoriented and drowsy."

S.N.   "They did become disoriented in a way. Paul tries to remember the details of the last people he saw and cannot. Mouchette sees old Menetriére, who for a moment seems real, who then disappears like a ghost."

S.N.   "Mouchette also hears a mixture of voices that become inhuman as she descends into the water."

S.N.   "When I was in high school I read *Anna Karenina* and, it seems to me that her suicide resembles Paul's and Mouchette's. It isn't only the losses that she endures which were terrible enough. She was denied association with her only son. And her lover, Vronsky, who begged her to leave her loveless marriage, leaves her without a word . . . just leaves a letter."

S.N.   "I read that, too. And, I remember that Russian society judged her and shunned her."

S.N.   "But, what I wanted to say was that her last moments of life were very similar to Mouchette's and Paul's. She had lost all that was dear to her and she was despairing. She leaves St. Petersburg on the evening train. At a stop along the way she leaves the train and wanders along the track becoming more and more disoriented. People didn't seem real to her. She is extremely exhausted and becomes drowsy just as they did. But, as Bernanos said, suicide isn't usually the conclusion of a supreme

> debate between the instinct to live and another, more mysterious instinct of renouncement and refusal. But it is not like that . . . suicide is an inexplicable and frighteningly sudden event, rather like the kind of rapid chemical decompositions which currently-fashionable science can only explain with absurd or contradictory hypotheses.
>
> *(Bernanos, 1966, p. 119)*

CONCLUSION

Students are already aware of the circumstances that are usually noted as those that place teenagers at risk for potential self-harm. Among these are a troubled home and school life, lack of meaningful communication with parents and peers, loss of a loved one, broken romance, sexual confusion, disciplinary crises, acquaintance with someone who has taken his or her life, mood disorder, and drug abuse. Here, students find these factors present in Mouchette and Paul's stories and other, more subtle reasons which ultimately lead to their suicides. Paul and Mouchette, in their underdeveloped states, possessed neither the resources of self-understanding nor the sophistication necessary to avoid abuse or to handle misdirected impulses. They were at the mercy of their community's indifference and of their own temperaments and age. Already at serious risk because of their tenuous positions in life, when they are stripped of their personal sense of pride and honor, they are thrust into a devastating emotional state that severs their anchor to life.

The Exile of Grief:
Mason, *Gilgamesh*

6

She made me see
Things as a man, and a man sees death in things
That is what it is to be a man. You'll know
When you have lost your strength to see
The way you once did. You'll be alone to wander
Looking for that life that's gone or some
Eternal life you have to find.
He drew closer to his friend's face.
My pain is that my eyes and ears
No longer see and hear the same
As yours do. Your eyes have changed.
You are crying. You never cried before.
It's not like you.
Why am I to die,
You to wander on alone?
Is that the way it is with friends?

Herbert Mason, 1972, p. 49

Portions of the précis appeared in *Clinical Nurse Specialist: The Journal for Advanced Nursing Practice*.

GILGAMESH

Gilgamesh, a retelling by Herbert Mason. New York: Mentor NAL, 1972. Copyright © 1970 Herbert Mason. Reprinted by permission of Houghton Mifflin Co. All rights reserved.

Names and Places Appearing in the Narrative

Anu (A'nu): The father of the Sumerian gods. The cosmic mountain, created from the primeval sea, had two parts: heaven (An) and earth (Ki), divided by the god Enlil, who proceeded to manage the affairs of the latter, with Anu overseeing the former. A temple in Uruk bore his name.

Bull of Heaven: Figure of drought created by Anu for Ishtar as a punishment for Gilgamesh's arrogance.

Ea (E'a): God of fresh springs; patron of the arts; friend of mankind.

Enkidu (En-ki'du): Friend of Gilgamesh; figure of natural man; patron saint of animals. A goddess of creation, Aruru, was supposed to have created him on the Steppe from clay in the image of Anu.

Enlil (En'lil): God of earth, wind, and spirit. He is merged in the present narrative with Ninurta, the war god.

Gilgamesh (Gil'ga-mesh): Fifth king of Uruk after the great flood; son of the goddess-prophetess Ninsun and a priest of Uruk. He is two-thirds god, one-third man, noted as a builder-King.

Humbaba (Hum-ba'ba): Guardian of the cedar forest; nature divinity; killed by Gilgamesh and Enkidu.

Ishtar (Ish'tar): Goddess of love and fertility, and of war; the daughter of Anu; patroness of Uruk.

Ishullanu (I'shul-la'nu): Anu's gardner; rejected by Ishtar, who turned him into a mole.

(Continued on page 132.)

CLASS DISCUSSION

Prior to class students closely read and annotated what they considered to be key passages to their understanding of this ancient epic story and its themes of friendship, grief, longing and the search for eternal life. During class discussion, they then highlighted their understanding of this story and its relevance to their lives and nursing practice. Class began with the following quote from Mason's *Gilgamesh*. Note the depth and variety of the responses as they unfold.

> *It is an old story*
> *But one that can still be told*
> *About a man who loved*
> *And lost his friend to death*
> *And learned he lacked the power*
> *To bring him back to life.*
> *It is the story of Gilgamesh*
> *And his friend Enkidu.*

Mason, 1972

S.N. "I did not have any sympathy for Gilgamesh in the beginning of this story. He was a callous bully. It's outrageous to think that he could just order his people about at whim."

S.N. "It's even more outrageous that he slept with all of the brides before their husbands."

S.N. "It's an ancient story . . . things are not that way today."

S.N. "There are things happening in the world today that parallel that behavior. Women still struggle against this sort of thing."

S.N. "As a man, he seems more like a teenager than a king. He can't make up his mind whether he wants to build walls or hang about doing nothing. He even lost interest in sleeping with the brides."

S.N. "He is a lonely man, lonely and bored."

S.N. "It is hard for me, or should I say, was hard for me to relate to this story at first. The names were so different and the places, well, I had to look them up to find out exactly where they were."

Mashu (Ma'shu): A mountain with twin peaks (the Lebanon ranges), behind which the sun descends at nightfall and out of which it rises at dawn.

Ninsun (Nin'sun): Mother of Gilgamesh; minor goddess known for wisdom.

Scorpion man and woman: Guardians of the entrance to Mashu.

Shamash (Sha'mash): The sun; husband and brother of Ishtar; son of Sin, the moon god.

Siduri (Sid-ur'i): Classic barmaid who lives by the sea.

Urshanabi (Ur'sha-na'bi): The boatman of Utnapishtim at the waters of the dead. His actual role in the epic, a subject of numerous scholarly studies and interpretations, is greatly reduced in this narrative.

Uruk (Ir'uk): Biblical Erech in southern Babylonia; seat of an important dynasty of kings following the flood.

Utnapishtim (Ut'na-pish-tim): Wise man of Shurrupak, one of the oldest cities of Mesopotamia, situated about twenty miles north of Uruk. His name means "He who saw life." He was protected from the flood by Ea.

(Mason, 1972, pp. 95–96)

Gilgamesh is an ancient Mesopotamian legend and epic poem dating from the third millennium B.C. which illuminates the themes of friendship and loss, and the search for eternal life. Here it is retold in the form of a verse narrative. The story of a god-like tyrant king (Gilgamesh) and an innocent, animal-like man (Enkidu) portrays the ways in which they become humanized together through their friendship. When Gilgamesh loses his fraternal companion in an unnecessary battle (which Gilgamesh contrived), he is nearly paralyzed by grief and longing for the first time in his life. His personal

(Continued on page 134.)

S.N. "I know what you mean, it's not only the names, but the idea of gods and goddesses, and god-like men and animal-like men. I didn't know what to make of all of it."

S.N. "Well, what is an epic poem anyway?"

S.N. "It's just a human story that has universal meaning. It has themes that have significance to everybody, you know, timeless."

S.N. "*Gilgamesh* does have important themes. I hadn't thought about friendship in just this way before. In the intensive care unit at the city hospital we had two teenagers that were in a car accident. They both had brain damage and a lot of other injuries. That was hard enough to cope with. But what blew me away was all of their friends. They kept coming and coming to the unit and they wandered around in a daze, or they sat and cried. It was overwhelming."

S.N. "I was on the unit then, too. And one of the things that I remember most was how bewildered they all seemed. It was as if they just could not believe that this happened to their friends."

S.N. "And while they had not died, the doctors told them that the two had sustained brain damage in the accident. They were in a coma and on life support."

S.N. "What this did, this accident, was to take away their world. Their world was not the same anymore. Everything was changed. The students couldn't function, they weren't going to school, they were drawn to the hospital like iron filings to a magnet."

S.N. "Yes, they almost seemed to think that somehow they would get some answers there. You know, why did it happen? What would happen to the two? How could they go on without them?"

S.N. "The story of Gilgamesh explains to me some of the things that happened during that month. Things that I didn't understand then. For one thing, I wanted to offer comfort to them and they just pushed me away, they wanted to be alone together. I was an outsider to them. And when the young girl, who was the passenger, died, the anger and crying was too much for me. I ended up sobbing myself and I didn't even know her. But even then, they turned away from me."

loss and passion to find the source of eternal life lifts him out of his indifference to human life, and he sets out on a journey to find a wise man, Utnapishtim, who was chosen by the old gods to survive the great flood and who knows the secret of immortality. The journey is replete with adventures that nearly crush the grieving king and reduce him to a solitary, suffering "everyman." When Gilgamesh crosses the sea of death and is befriended by the aged and wise survivor, Utnapishtim, who has grieved over the multitude of losses from the flood, he is given the secret plant of eternal life. Renewed by the plant and excited by the prospect of living forever, he pauses to bathe in a pool, setting the plant aside. A serpent (nature itself), then rises from the water and devours the plant, leaving it behind as slough. This final loss reveals the journey's ultimate meaning for the young king: wisdom can only be attained by his facing his own mortality.

S.N.   "In this story the battle that Gilgamesh creates is one that didn't need to happen. And it's in that battle with the monster and then the Bull of Heaven that Enkidu is fatally wounded."

S.N.   "But, let's go back to what it was that made Gilgamesh and Enkidu good friends in the first place. I don't see evidence for such a deep friendship that would explain such sorrow."

S.N.   "I think that it does. Even if Gilgamesh is like a teenager, and Enkidu runs with the animals, they are capable of having a friendship."

S.N.   "But what is it based upon?"

S.N.   "First, competitiveness. They heard about one another. Enkidu did not like what he heard that Gilgamesh was doing with the brides. And, Gilgamesh was threatened by Enkidu's talents."

S.N.   "Then they met and had a hell of a fight, wore themselves out, and realized that they were alike."

S.N.   "I think that they realized that each complemented the other."

S.N.   "That's how the friendship began."

S.N.   "Then, they became inseparable. They vowed to each other that they would never be separated."

S.N.   "Teenagers make pledges like that."

S.N.   "Adults do, too, but, maybe the vow is not declared, it might be more silent."

S.N.   "This was the first real friendship for either Gilgamesh or Enkidu."

S.N.   "That makes it important."

S.N.   "Gilgamesh decides that they should do something noble together and that something is to kill the monster, Humbaba, the nature divinity, guardian of the cedar forest."

S.N.   "It isn't necessary for them to do this, why does Gilgamesh press so?"

S.N.   "Yes, he doesn't listen to the fears of his good friend, Enkidu. Enkidu thinks that it is they that will die instead."

S.N.   "Enkidu is an awesome guy, and he has a lot of power."

S.N.   "Gilgamesh takes his idea to the old generals and they get all excited over the possibilities. They encourage the young men to go on and battle Humbaba."

S.N.　"They are just like the older men that we have in government today who send the young off to war. They get all excited about it, you can see it on TV."

S.N.　"Politicians today think things out far more carefully than these men did."

S.N.　"I don't know, it seems as though everyone that they knew thought the battle was a great idea."

S.N.　"Gilgamesh's mother, Ninsun, didn't. And she was a minor goddess. known for her wisdom. She could interpret dreams. Gilgamesh relied on her to interpret his dreams."

S.N.　"She is the one who predicted from his dream that Enkidu would become important to him. He would 'lift him out of his tiredness.'"

S.N.　"Ninsun was afraid for her son and she asked Enkidu to protect him from Humbaba's anger."

S.N.　"Gilgamesh has this need for power and control. He has to show that he is more powerful than the worst guy around. He picks the fight. Humbaba did not come looking for them."

S.N.　"No, it's true, they provoked him into the fight."

S.N.　"At this point Gilgamesh doesn't take the idea of death very seriously. Whereas Enkidu is truly scared."

S.N.　"That's because Gilgamesh never lost anyone, maybe Enkidu saw death in nature a lot."

S.N.　"There's another thing, Gilgamesh gets pleasure out of fear and danger."

S.N.　"Fear separated them then, because Enkidu has the exact opposite reaction:

Enkidu was alone
With sights he saw brought on by pain
And fear, as one in deep despair
May lie beside his love who sleeps
And seems so unafraid, absorb in himself the
*　　phantoms*
That she cannot see—phantoms diminished for one
When two can see and stay awake to talk of them
And search out a solution to despair,
Or lie together in each other's arms,
Or weep and in exhaustion from their tears

Perhaps find laughter fro their fears.
But alone and awake the size and nature
Of the creatures in his mind grow monstrous.

(Mason, 1972, p. 36)

S.N.   "Look at the great difference in the way these two approach this battle. Gilgamesh is strutting about, can't wait to get at it. He isn't fully a friend yet if he can say what he did to Enkidu knowing full well how terrorized he is:

> *Why are you worried about death?*
> *Only the gods are immortal anyway,*
> *Sighed Gilgamesh.*
> *What men do is nothing, so fear is never*
> *Justified. What happened to your power*
> *That once could challenge and equal mine?*
> *I will go ahead of you, and if I die*
> *I will at least have the reward*
> *Of having people say: He died in war*
> *Against Humbaba.*

(Mason, 1972, pp. 29, 30)

S.N.   "This is a good example of why hearing, really hearing another's fears is so important. Because patients do have great fears of treatments, diagnostic tests and the like. We don't share the same fear, but we should be ready to hear theirs in ways similar to what is suggested here.

> *When two can see and stay awake to talk of them*
> *And search out a solution to despair*

(Mason, 1972, p. 36)

S.N.   "When Gilgamesh strikes the cedar and Humbaba comes roaring at them, it is frightening. Even Gilgamesh is scared, so scared he can't move when Humbaba first attacks Enkidu. And I mean attacks, he nearly crushes him."

S.N.   "But, finally, Gilgamesh strikes out and cuts off Humbaba's head. This sounds like *Kagamusha* or something."

S.N.   "I am not familiar with all of these gods and goddesses but at this point the goddess of fertility, Ishtar, appears and sets to work on Gilgamesh, trying to win him for herself."

S.N.   "Yes, but all along in this tale, you will notice that Gilgamesh never stays long with the women. He is driven to go on this journey and even at this point before Enkidu is struck down, he doesn't want to linger. He actually is very insulting."

S.N.   "So Ishtar retaliates and sends the Bull of Heaven after Gilgamesh."

S.N.   "This time, Enkidu saves Gilgamesh, despite the wound inflicted by Humbaba."

S.N.   "Gilgamesh has insight for the first time of what it would mean to lose his friend:

> *I can't imagine being left alone,*
> *I'm less a man without my friend*

> (Mason, 1972, p. 47)

S.N.   "You see denial of the reality here, too:

> *Gilgamesh did not let himself believe*
> *The gods had chosen one of them to die.*

> (Mason, 1972, p. 47)

S.N.   "Gilgamesh wonders if he can reverse the god's decision, or should he relieve Enkidu's pain, he doesn't yet realize that he cannot reverse Enkidu's fate."

S.N.   "I have heard people plead with God not to take their relative. I heard some young parents praying just like that. I think that right up to the moment of death you have this hope that the person won't die. You pray for it not to happen."

S.N.   "When Gilgamesh does realize that Enkidu is dying he tries to recollect their life together, their life that was 'so empty of gesture they never felt they had to make' (Mason, 1972, p. 48). To me this means that they were so close they didn't have to talk about how close they were. They just knew, they trusted one another, they did not have to prove their loyalty to one another over and over again."

S.N.   "Enkidu seems so wise in his last words, he is so human, and he is worried for the friend he is leaving. Their life together as friends was far different than if they had never met."

S.N.   "That's for sure. Enkidu would never have provoked Humbaba on his own. He would still be alive in this tale."

S.N.   "But what I think he is saying is that both were changed because they had this friendship. He laments what has happened to him and also what will happen to Gilgamesh whom he knows will miss him terribly. Death is a cruel thing."

S.N.   "Gilgamesh is responsible for the whole thing from beginning to end. It was he who sent the prostitute to humanize Enkidu in the forest. And we all know what happened once the two men met. Enkidu would never have come to the city, Uruk, if he had not become less wild, if he had never heard of Gilgamesh."

S.N.   "He knows what he is talking about in his parting words to Gilgamesh. And he, too, wants to recount how they came to be together. He's less sentimental than Gilgamesh, he says very straightforwardly:

> *She made me see*
> *Things as a man, and a man sees death in things.*
> *That is what it is to be a man. You'll know*
> *When you have lost the strength to see*
> *The way you once did. You'll be alone and wander*
> *Looking for that life that's gone or some*
> *Eternal life you have to find.*
> *He drew closer to his friend's face.*
> *My pain is that my eyes and ears*
> *No longer see and hear the same*
> *As yours do. Your eyes have changed.*
> *You are crying. You never cried before.*
> *It's not like you.*
> *Why am I to die,*
> *You to wander on alone?*
> *Is that the way it is with friends?*

(Mason, 1972, pp. 49, 50)

S.N.   "Yes, he is telling Gilgamesh, 'a man sees death in things.' That's reality, people do die, those who love them have to go on. But, he is feeling great sorrow for himself and for his friend. He knows that his friend, who has never lost anyone that he loved before, will have a very difficult time after he is dead."

S.N.   "This is the first time that he has seen Gilgamesh deeply affected by the possibility of losing him. Isn't it amazing that he is dying and yet his concern is for his friend. I think that is a deep, lasting friendship."

S.N.   "What Enkidu says will happen to Gilgamesh describes exactly what happened to me. I felt just that way when I lost my high school friend. I was different, everyone else was different. No one measured up anymore. My friend and I did everything together, shared all our secrets, planned to go off to college together. I never, ever, imagined a world without her in it. I cried all of the time. I felt totally changed. Every time I read this passage, I cry. This happened four years ago, but I am always seeing something that I think she will like, or something I want to share with her. And then, when I remember that I can't, I have this awful empty feeling."

S.N.   "I had another reaction, I'm a bit older than you, but when I was in high school, I had a pal that died. I guess I tried to deny how important she was to me, didn't even go to the funeral. But reading this story brought it all back, it seems like it just happened yesterday, like no time had gone by at all."

S.N.   "That makes me appreciate the importance of friendship all the more. We hear a lot in our classes about families, but not much about the implications of friendship. This deserves more thought."

S.N.   "What is friendship, do you think?"

S.N.   "Why is it so different than other relationships?"

S.N.   "It has something to do with caring about someone because you have something in common. You develop in it. I don't know, but it's different than being with brothers or sisters, or other relatives. You might be close to family members, but partly that's because you are related, you have to have some kind of closeness to them."

S.N. "I think that I'm different, a different person with my friends than with relatives. I feel more like myself, not like someone's niece or sister or daughter. Not that I don't think that relatives aren't important or that I don't love them. But, somehow, I feel different with my close friends. Maybe I feel freer?"

S.N. "I can understand, in part, what you are saying about the difference between being with friends and relatives. I feel that way, too, with the exception of my time spent with my grandmothers. I felt very free with them."

S.N. "But there is the difference of generations there."

S.N. "I think that age has nothing to do with it, there can be a big difference in the ages of friends. You don't have to be the exact age as your friends. You might be in school, but by the time you are an adult, your friends are any age."

S.N. "Even when you are young, friends are any age."

S.N. "But, what exactly is a friend? It isn't enough to say that it is someone you share troubles or secrets with. Or even someone that you do things with."

S.N. "Friends are more companions, people that you don't have to explain yourself to, you can just be with them."

S.N. "I think friends are people who are always straight with you, if they see you getting in trouble, they will talk to you about it, they won't help you look the other way."

S.N. "Maybe friends are more spiritual companions than other people in your life. You know, you share ideas and hopes with them, things of the mind."

S.N. "How do Enkidu and Gilgamesh fit into these descriptions?"

S.N. "They did everything together. And they shared their fears with one another."

S.N. "They depended on one another, not in the same way that they depended on Gilgamesh's mother."

S.N. "They became a part of one another. They were different, more complete because of their friendship. And that is why Gilgamesh is so devastated when Enkidu dies. It isn't just that he has never lost anyone before, that is too simple an answer, and his grief is too big for that to be the explanation."

S.N. "Yes, he is losing his dear friend, and he is losing part of himself, somehow."

S.N.   "Gilgamesh is really stricken with grief, and he is angry and bitter, just like what was talked about in class today.

> *Gilgamesh wept bitterly for his friend*
> *He felt himself now singled out for loss*
> *Apart from everyone else. The word Enkidu*
> *Roamed through every thought*
> *Like a hungry animal through empty lairs*
> *In search of food. The only nourishment*
> *He knew was grief, endless in its hidden source*
> *Yet never ending hunger.*

(Mason, 1972, p. 53)

S.N.   "It is as though the grief takes over your whole self like some awful illness. It affects your every thought, the way you feel physically, everything."

S.N.   "It colors your whole world. You feel like an alien everywhere you go. You can't even sleep the way you once did. In a way, you are possessed."

S.N.   "I know that I didn't want anyone to intrude on what I was thinking even. And everything reminded me of her, so even if I wasn't thinking of her for a few minutes, someone would say something or I would see something that would trigger thoughts of her.'"

S.N.   "I got very angry at someone who pressed me to talk about my friend."

S.N.   "Why?"

S.N.   "I wanted her all to myself. I did not want to share what we had with anyone."

S.N.   "I had never thought about grief the way that we have talked about here. The notion that 'Grief is endless in its hidden source' is very, very different than the way I had grief explained in my own mind. But I think that grief is like that, otherwise it would begin and end like a bout of flu or something, it would be totally predictable."

S.N.   "And we have said today that it was still active four years later. Also, that it has an endless source. Once a person has this experience, this grief happens, it is a natural thing. You can try to escape it but it crops up later anyway."

S.N.   "We have learned in other classes that if it is denied it can affect thinking and health for years. And it can lead to other illnesses because it is unresolved."

S.N.   "But that makes it sound time limited. In this story there is an evolution in Gilgamesh, but only after he goes through a lot of torment."

S.N.   "He is not in a position to meet another friend at this time."

S.N.   "Some might hope that another new friend might come along so that they could have some relief from thinking about the one that they lost."

S.N.   "In our story, Gilgamesh never felt so alone, he wandered in the desert. I suppose that some might say he was mad because he dressed up in animal skins and threw himself into the dust."

S.N.   "But don't you see? Enkidu was an animal-like man and Gilgamesh wanted to literally be him, to keep him alive this way. I don't think it is uncommon at all. My grandmother saved all of my grandfather's favorite things, all of his tools, and every bit of his clothes. Once, when I went over to visit, she was wearing one of his flannel shirts."

S.N.   "What he is really up to is trying to find some way to bring Enkidu back to life and wearing the skins, or your grandmother wearing the flannel shirt makes them feel a little closer to their lost friend and husband."

S.N.   "I can accept that all right, but I have a lot of trouble with finding the source of eternal life. You can't bring people back to life. And I don't believe there is life anywhere else but here. When they are dead, they are gone."

S.N.   "But maybe even back then, 4000 years ago, they were concerned about whether or not there was an after-life. Maybe they hoped that there was. Otherwise, why would they be so knowledgeable about grief?"

S.N.   "Right, remember, this story was sort of cast in stone in cuneiform writing. It was only discovered in the middle of the last century."

S.N.   "The tablets also described Gilgamesh looking for Utnapishtim because he was considered a wise man who it was thought could help Gilgamesh in his search."

S.N.   "But, at first, Gilgamesh doesn't expect help from anyone and I wondered why that was. We have learned that it is important to try to help comfort people who have lost a loved one. I never, ever, expected that they might not want it, or wouldn't expect it."

S.N.   "This may be similar to the teenagers in the intensive care unit, they separated themselves from the hospital staff, and their parents for the most part. They clung together. It was almost as though they wanted to be alone together, but now I am thinking that maybe they didn't think that anyone of us could help them with the dreadful feelings they were having."

S.N.   "It's possible that they had no expectation of ever feeling anything else."

S.N.   "This reminds me of a cousin of mine, who, on the day of his father's funeral, got incredibly upset with his aunts who were trying to comfort him. He was furious with the joking and laughing that was going on at the wake. He told me he resented it, it was an insult to his father."

S.N.   "It sounds like it was an insult to him, too."

S.N.   "I remember going to my uncle's funeral, when I tried to hug my aunt and tell her how sorry I was, she looked at me like she didn't know me."

S.N.   "She must have been in shock like Watanabe was the day he learned that he was fatally ill."

S.N.   "People do wonder if there is an after-life. I'm afraid that someone is going to ask me about it and I won't know what to say to them."

S.N.   "Well, in this story, we sure do get different points of view on that subject."

S.N.   "First of all there are the Scorpion people, the ones who guard Mashu. These are the first that Gilgamesh meets on his journey. They are afraid of human feelings, they only see death as a possibility. They certainly do not have any hope for life after death."

S.N.   "It's safe to say that a large segment of the population has similar beliefs. What makes this crucial to know about is that what they think, if they are the doctor or nurse or counselor for the dying, their beliefs may color the grief of that person."

S.N.   "Yes, don't forget the doctor and nurse in *Ikiru*. The nurse said that if she learned that she had only 6 months to live, she would take poison."

S.N.   "That doesn't mean that she does, or doesn't believe in an after-life."

S.N.   "No, maybe not, but it does indicate a certain lack of hope."

S.N.   "I think that what we think about these things, or should I say what we believe, what we value, is transmitted to our patients. Think of this, if we were afraid of human feelings they certainly would know."

S.N.   "You would have to have a real dialogue going on actively with your patient, otherwise you wouldn't be of any help at all."

S.N.   "Explain that, won't you?"

S.N.   "I just mean that we are present for the dying and their relatives and we want to make the death as reasonable as possible. You can't know what that will be unless you are in a dialogue with the people involved. They will be flooded with all kinds of emotion and they may want to be alone, they might need comfort. I guess I just mean that there is not one single thing that is just the right thing to say or do. That can only emerge in what you do together."

S.N.   "This, in part, could explain why Gilgamesh left Siduri, the barmaid who took him in when he was exhausted and half starved. He looks so crazed that she is afraid of him, but then she pities him. She has imagined that she knows what he needs without asking him. He needs physical comforts, a cozy home life, good food, her charms."

S.N.   "But, when she tells Gilgamesh to 'put this behind you, go on' and then, 'the gods gave death to man, you just have to accept it' (Mason, 1972, p. 65), Gilgamesh feels like he is suffocating."

S.N.   "That is because he didn't want to forget his friend, that's only logical."

S.N.   "There are nurses and doctors who say very similar things. It's the 'come on, let's get going' philosophy."

S.N.   "When Gilgamesh rejects Siduri, she is furious and she tells him that he 'is filled with love of self and rage.' That means, to me, that she is insulted because he doesn't like her solutions to his grief."

S.N.   "That is because she was offering her personal self as a solution."

S.N.   "She was also giving advice to someone who was taken over by a grief that they wanted. That sounds odd, but the grief made him feel close to Enkidu."

S.N.   "So, he would think that she was telling him that she would be a substitute for Enkidu, take his place in Gilgamesh's affections."

S.N.   "They part in a rage. And then he goes to the shore and smashes the precious stones that he needs to continue his journey."

S.N.   "He strikes out at everything. He reminds me of my cousin here, too. After he blew up at my aunts, he went up to his room and tore it apart."

S.N.   "You know, there are a lot of physical symptoms that are mentioned in this story, too, the fact that grief causes a tightness in the chest, this kind of anger, and an unending fatigue."

S.N.   "All the while he continues on his journey, frightfully alone. He can't see beside him or in front of him on the Road of the Sun. He is as totally isolated as a human can be. He only has his grief for company. He must have felt waves of emptiness and fear, and he comforted himself by whispering over and over again, 'Enkidu, Enkidu.' Imagine being so alone."

S.N.   "And what first brings him out of it is great beauty, the Valley of the Precious Stones. When he sees it, he is 'overcome with pain.' And he has a deep longing for his friend:

> *Gazing into the valley*
> *He felt overcome with pain*
> *As a man*
> *Who has been in prison*
> *Feels his chains*
> *At release from fear.*
> *He spoke Enkidu's name aloud*

(Mason, 1972, p. 60)

S.N.   "The great beauty could be for others, music, or a painting, or something in nature, that could stir someone who is grieving."

S.N.   "This is the first that he is able to voice his sorrow but afterwards he feels more alone and openly weeps."

S.N.   "It is after this that he meets Siduri who then sends him to Urshanabi, the boatman of the Waters of the Dead."

S.N.   "Urshanabi wants Gilgamesh to tell him why he looks so wasted but Gilgamesh refuses, he doesn't want to retell his pain. But when he says he only wants to bring Enkidu back to life, once again he lapses into telling of his great loss."

S.N.   "But there is a difference now because he realized he does not want to hear this any longer, he has come too far on his search, his journey, to go on with retelling. Now he wants to find release from his despair."

S.N.   "Urshanabi actually tells him that his presence is exhausting to others. He moralizes at Gilgamesh and acts like he has the answer to his troubles. But he accuses him of being selfish, for wanting what no other person has been able to have . . . the power to bring someone back to life."

S.N.   "He does tell Gilgamesh how to get across the Sea of Death to the wise man, Utnapishtim, who was welcoming to him."

S.N.   "Yes, I noticed that he was so, sort of benevolent looking, that Gilgamesh felt the first relief he had experienced since his friend died. It must have been in the man's manner and his appearance, this calmness."

S.N.   "Gilgamesh asks him beseechingly,

Is that something more than death?
Some other end to friendship?

(Mason, 1972, p. 73)

S.N.   "He sounds like Ivan Ilych, doesn't he? 'Where will I be when I am no more?' (Tolstoi, 1960, p. 130)."

S.N.   "It's the big question, isn't it?"

S.N.   "Utnapishtim understands the question and tells him that he is impressed that he would come that far. Now he must borrow light from the blind. I think that means that he knows he is sincere, and that his answer can only come from someone who sees beyond despair, beyond ordinary things."

S.N.   "Despair isn't ordinary."

S.N.   "What he suggests is that there is more than despair. You have to have faith that it is there, you can't see it, it isn't tangible."

S.N.   "Utnapishtim talks about the love of a friend in a way full of wisdom:

> *Friendship is vowing towards immortality*
> *Does not know the passing away of beauty*
> *(Though take care!)*
> *Because it aims for the spirit*
> *Many years ago through loss I learned*
> *That love is wrung from our inmost heart*
> *Until only the loved one is and we are not.*

(Mason, 1972, p. 74)

S.N.   "I'm not sure that I understand what this means."

S.N.   "To me it says that deep love, like the love of these two friends, is immortal."

S.N.   "Well, Gilgamesh doesn't understand this because he still wants some magical word or a gesture that will give him back his friend, something he can actually see."

S.N.   "Utnapishtim tells him about the sacred plant on the river bottom. Gilgamesh dives down to the bottom with the help of stones he ties to his feet and finds this plant. But, then, he carelessly leaves it on the river bank while he is swimming and a snake eats it. What does this all mean?"

S.N.   "This plant exists, but it is not for mortals to hold."

S.N.   "Gilgamesh is truly sad when he discovers how careless he was, but by this time he knows with a certainty that he has gone as far as he can go. And I think he feels different. He doesn't try to share his story any longer. He has accepted that he cannot bring his friend back to life."

S.N.   "When he returns to Uruk, he notices new walls that his people have built in his absence. And he doesn't have this urge to tell of his loss to others as you said."

S.N.   "But he still feels a sadness."

S.N.   "Perhaps he will bring back to his people this wisdom that he has gained on his long, long journey. He can help them with their losses because of what he faced."

S.N.   "Then he will have become an honorable leader and very much unlike the one he was in the beginning, lazing about, bored, sleeping with other men's wives for amusement."

S.N.   "He has become more sensitive to others because of his grief. His grief made him aware of his own capacity for deep feelings."

S.N.   "For me, this means that he is a changed man who will not treat any other living thing in a cavalier manner ever again."

S.N.   "All of this is true because he now actually knows what being connected to another costs."

CONCLUSION

Through this ancient Sumerian epic poem one can see that the pain and mystery of loss is shared by man and woman throughout time. When one realizes that death is a possibility, one discovers solitude, the importance of others, and the question of life beyond death. When one loses a loved one, one never sees or hears the world the same again. This world seen through the eyes of grief seems barren and desolate. But grief can also mysteriously strengthen and give hope in ways unknown before.

As the students studied Gilgamesh they gained a fresh appreciation for the many facets of grief. They discussed the insights they had about the ways in which grief has affected them and those they have known. Especially noteworthy is the phenomena of grief as a necessary exile after the loss of a loved one. In their desire to become of assistance to the grieving they feel a kinship with Gilgamesh, who, after his long journey, searching for the source of eternal life, comes home to Uruk a changed man. He is a more sensitive man who no longer treats others cavalierly. As one student said, "He has become more sensitive to others because of his grief."

Nurses experience loss in great measure and they are not "immune to these deep sorrows" (Young-Mason, 1991, p. 122). A fuller understanding of the depth of sorrow and a "grief . . . endless in its hidden source" (Mason, 1972, p. 53) offers nurses consolation for the losses they endure. Further, when the journey through grief is valued, mysteriously, hope can emerge.

In the following short stories, two young student nurses face sudden loss and grief for the first time. The losses are different for one of these two babies survives, but with a destroyed mind. The other dies of SIDS inexplicably while the mother is in the next room putting another child to bed. The students lose an accustomed sense of well being as they face these devastating losses. They are left with the haunting reminder that young infants can be harmed and that they can die suddenly. In this new vulnerability, the students become sensitive to their own pain and that of those around them.

First Encounter with Death
Hwayun Lee

It's my first day at the Pediatric Intensive Care Unit just to observe. There was minimum activity yesterday. They had only one patient who has been there for six months. "Oh! They have a new patient who came in this morning. He's a SIDS baby? Isn't that sudden infant death syndrome? Let's look it up."

> There is no known etiology but it causes death to infants of 1 month to 1 year old. However, an infant cannot be identified with a SIDS without an autopsy first.

"I guess that's why his chart reads 'S/P Respiratory Arrest.' I wonder if I could go and look at the baby. Ohh . . . he's such an adorable, chubby baby. He looks just like a big doll. Why is there blood all over his legs and the bed? It looks awful. I wish we could clean it up."

"Who is this? It must be their family minister who came in to support the family. Wait . . . I think he's crying. He isn't allowed to cry, is he? Isn't he supposed to be the strong one? What did he say? 'The baby looks so helpless.' "Yeah, I can see that, but I thought death wasn't a sad event because we return to our Maker, our God. Oh my goodness, I'm not going to cry. There is no need to be sad. Nope, death is just part of life and we need to accept that. Right?"

"Here comes the mother. She's thin and she looks awfully tired. It doesn't look like she is handling this very well. I wonder if when I become a mother I could handle it. I wish I could give her a hug, but, better not."

"Wow, the charge nurse is so under control. She's giving the baby a bath and making his crib up. This feels good, helping the nurse to wash the blood from the baby's legs. I need to get a clean johnny from the pediatric unit. Hmmm, it feels good to leave the PICU. I didn't realize how stuffy it was in there."

"The baby looks good now, washed up, in a clean johnny in a clean crib."

"Here comes the physician. Whoa, he is so confusing! He's describing to the family what is happening to the baby. He seems too impersonal! Look, doctor! Can't you see that the mother is not even listening? She's just standing there beside the father, staring at their baby. I wonder what she is thinking. Why does my heart feel so heavy?"

"There goes the physician. I guess he finally realized the parents weren't listening to him. Wait, is that him out there talking to the residents in the hall? Why can't he go somewhere else? Doesn't he know that we can hear him in here through these open sliding doors? Even though the parents seem oblivious to what's happening around them, it could be annoying that the physician has more to say and it's not to them. Good. I'm so glad the nurse closed the doors. I guess I could have done the same."

"I think the mother finally realizes Samuel is not going home with her. Although she keeps saying that he looks much better here at the hospital than when she found him in his crib. Why is she thinking of the things she did wrong last night? She says after putting him to sleep, she stepped out of his room to put his little sister to bed. When she returned to check on Samuel, she found him at the corner of the crib, not breathing, turning blue. I wish someone would tell her that she didn't do anything wrong. It's actually difficult to identify any cause of SIDS."

"She finally wants to hold him, even though, at first, she is afraid of the tubes and lines attached to her son. This is so beautiful. Better leave and give the family some privacy. Oh! This really stinks! Death can be so cruel. Especially when there is no reason for it, no explanation and no warning. He's so little. I wish there was something we could do."

"Oh, the father came out of the unit. I wonder if he needs anything or if he is looking for someone. Everyone seems busy." "Can I help you?" "He only wants a box of tissues. I can get that for him. It's time for me to leave. I wish I could stay a bit longer; this is as close as I have come to death. But, now it's time for my post clinical conference."

"It's my turn to present. 'Today, the PICU had a SIDS baby who came in at 4 O' Clock this morning. This is my first encounter with death. He looked so . . . ' What's the matter with me? Why can't I talk anymore? Why am I crying?"

Haunting Screams
by Lisa Smith

The young student nurse who stepped off the elevator on her way to the Pediatric Unit had no idea of what lay ahead for her that afternoon. So far her assignments in the pediatric clinical rotation had been older children and teenagers. Every week she hoped that she would be given an infant to care for, but she was always disappointed. "I'll probably get another teenager again today. I'm tired of this!" she complained to her friend as they hurried down the hall.

Suddenly her very being was pierced with the awful sound of a baby in excruciating pain. It was like nothing she had ever heard before; it was more like screaming than crying. Then she realized that the screaming was coming from a baby held in her instructor's arms.

"What's wrong, little one? Why are you so upset?" the student said as she gently stroked the baby's brow.

"This is Katiana," said the clinical instructor, "she needs someone to be patient, someone to give her lots of love. That's going to be your job! This little munchkin is yours today!"

"Oh, great!" the student said, trying to sound enthusiastic and confident. Inside she was trembling with excitement and fear.

The baby looked scary the way her back arched and her arms and legs flailed about. Between screams her tongue protruded out and her eyes darted randomly back and forth as if she were watching a fly buzz around her head.

"Go and read the Kardex and her chart and then come back and take her from me," said the instructor. "You aren't going to have much to do except to try to feed her and bathe her. Your main task is to try and calm her down. And that's not going to be easy!"

"Oh, great!" the student thought again with some dismay. In the mass confusion of the Nurses' Station she began to read through the child's medical record. She wasn't prepared for what she found. The diagnosis was multiple subdural hematoma. Now the student nurse understood why the baby looked the way she did. And as she read on her mouth began to gape open. Katiana had been brought to the Emergency Room by her mother who claimed that ever since the child had fallen out of her playpen she had been acting strange. Through a CT Scan the doctors had discovered not just one hematoma but multiple ones all over the brain. Clearly she did not just "fall out of her playpen."

The student nurse could barely hear Katiana's screams over the buzzing in her head. Her stomach wrenched tight with anger as she read on. "Abuse" it said. Katiana's parents were being brought up on charges of child abuse. The student stared at the medical record page. She felt overwhelmed. The words became fuzzy as she tried to picture what happened in her mind. She saw the mother standing over the crying baby in the playpen and . . . .

"Excuse me, could I borrow Katiana's chart for a minute?" asked a doctor.

"Oh, yeah, sure. Here you go," she said nervously handing over the chart to a doctor with a name pin that said "Department of Neurology." She felt foolish being caught daydreaming.

Then she returned to her clinical instructor and Katiana. Somehow the baby looked different to her. She didn't seem scary anymore. As she took Katiana from her instructor's arms she was flooded with a jumble of emotions. At first she felt nervous and awkward, afraid that she might hurt the baby if she held her wrong. Katiana was screaming so loud it was hard not to think she was causing her pain. As she walked down the hall towards Katiana's room she could see people turn their heads to look at them. Finally they reached the room. She went straight to the rocking chair in the corner and sat down with the child in her arms.

"Shh! Shh! It's OK. You're OK now. Nobody's going to hurt you, I promise!" the student said as she tried to get comfortable. But this was impossible. Katiana arched her back so hard that she couldn't hold her any other way but to cradle her, and when she did that her head pushed so hard into the student's forearm it made red marks. The young nurse finally gave up trying to get comfortable. She rocked in the chair and sang softly to the child who continued to scream uncontrollably.

The student looked closer at the shrieking child in her arms. She was such a beautiful little baby. Her skin was a soft light brown and on top of her head was a big clump of coal black hair. When she opened her little pink mouth to scream, the student could see all the way back to her throat.

"What a loud one you are!" she said.

Slowly the child began to quiet down. The student's heart ached as she looked at the baby's innocent face. She looked into her big brown eyes, they were blankly staring. It was as if the child had shut herself off from the world because she had been hurt so badly. The young student nurse looked away so as to distract herself, tears trickled down her cheeks. Looking at the child's eyes this way made the reality of the whole situation hit her hard. "How could a woman bring such a beautiful creature into the world only to shake all of the life out of her?" the student wondered. She's never going to be normal again and they probably don't even care.

The student's arm was killing her but she didn't want to move because the baby was finally quiet. She started to think about the mother again and wondered why she would do such an awful thing. "She must have a terrible life herself to do something like this. She had to have been really desperate. Maybe she was doing drugs or drinking, or maybe she was beaten herself. Maybe all of life's pressures just got to her so bad that she was out of control. Maybe she couldn't stop herself." But none of these excuses made the student feel any better about the helpless child she held in her arms. It just didn't make any sense at all.

For those eight hours she held little Katiana in her arms. She went round and round with these thoughts, sometimes frustrated, sometimes angry, but most of all, deeply saddened that this child would be immeasurably wounded and, alas, it happens all of the time. She had read and also heard about child abuse hundreds of times. But it had always been something that seemed so awful it was unreal. Katiana was real. Her pain and suffering were undeniably real. The student nurse wanted to take the pain and suffering away from her so badly, but she couldn't, and this made her feel powerless and frustrated.

When it came time to leave, she was exhausted. "OK sweetheart, I have to go now, but don't worry, the nurses will take great care of you," she whispered to the little girl as she kissed her on the forehead. Her arms ached with fatigue when she handed her over to the next nurse. The relief she felt in her arms she wished she could feel in her heart. Her head began to throb. She walked away from the little child whose screaming had begun again. Slowly she gathered her things and walked to the elevator as the unit doors shut out the child's haunting screams.

Conclusion

Selected works of Sophocles, Tolstoi, Bernanos, Cather, Kurosawa, Mason, and Rodin were studied within this course to foster a deeper understanding of suffering and compassion. The depictions of Philoctetes, Ivan Ilych, Mouchette and Paul, Watanabe, Gilgamesh and the Burghers, through their exile, taught the students that compassion can only be understood through action. Compassion, like freedom, is a word whose meaning becomes clearer and finally clarified in practice, when known through desire and need, in hands-on life, so to speak. Also, like freedom, compassion is shown to be a mutual act drawn from interdependence between two or more people who suffer together for its realization. While freedom may seem an individual experience demanding that an individual act his or her way out of passivity, it, in fact, depends on action and reaction from others to be realized or denied. Compassion is also an action and a reaction, an interchange of desires which form a passion in which one takes on and gives and another gives and takes on. That action diminishes the isolation and passivity that can exaggerate suffering beyond a human being's capacity to endure and even psychologically control its passage through his or her body and psyche. This interchange is most profoundly and vividly depicted in works of literature and art which mirror human life in its range of experiences, especially its passions and extreme capacities, its release and suffering, its cravings for freedom and needs of compassion. No text book can express the simple unselfconscious, monosyllabic cry of pain and joy found in life and echoed in literature, which goes deeper than any theory about humanity can. Thus, literature is a crucial primary source for those concerned about human care, especially for those needing to deepen their understanding of how humans both need and are aroused to give care. It is a mirror that shows both career and cared for sharing in the action of compassion, through their common humanity responding in each.

Notes to Teachers and Students

It should be apparent to the reader that this text is not aimed at literary criticism in any way. Rather, it is an exploration of the correspondences between art and literature and nursing phenomena meant to deepen and fortify student nurses for their future practice. This explains, in part, why this exploration should be conducted by a nurse educator and not an English teacher who would, by nature and training, seek to critique and interpret literary works toward another end. The nurse educator does not necessarily attempt to interpret style and language, but rather concentrates on what the art and fiction reveals of the human condition, specifically the ways in which values, beliefs, and spirituality affect behavior, health, and healing. Further, the nurse educator has experienced hands-on care of others in deep psychological and physical need. She or he is acculturated to the development of knowledge in the profession as it speaks to the human response of the experience of illness. Finally, the daily experience of the world of the ill, the disfigured, and the dying places the nurse educator and the student nurse in the unique position of needing this dialogue both as enrichment and inner fortification.

Teachers and students who have not studied art and literature in relation to nursing phenomena before might like to begin this exploration with a specific methodology. For this the following guide might be of service. Essentially, what is of interest is the reasons for and the ways in which the character's passions, emotions, beliefs, and personal character traits affect his or her behavior and well being. To tease out the particulars then one would attempt to:

1. Dissect the ways in which the subjective experience (moral and personal) affects the individual.
2. Discern the individual's relation to objects, events, and other persons.
3. Explore the meaning of illness (somatic, psychiatric, spiritual) to the individual.
4. Study the way in which the body is viewed in the context of everyday life and function.
5. Demonstrate the manner in which the human consciousness is embodied.
6. Discover the impact of apperceptive reasoning.
7. Comprehend the meaning of human spirituality and its relation to behavior, health, and healing.

Following are essay questions which further assist in the exploration of the works discussed in this text.

Rodin, "The Burghers of Calais"

1. Who are the "Burghers of Calais?"
2. What was Rodin attempting to accomplish with his sculpture?
3. Why is their story of self-sacrifice important to know about?
4. What is Rodin's conception of "fugitive truth" and why is it important to know about in the representation of emotional states?
5. How is it that all aspects of the body convey emotion?
6. Explain the ways in which the Burghers represent the emotions that people experience when facing death.

Kurosawa, *Ikiru*

1. Describe Mr. Watanabe as a young father.
2. How did he become an institutional bureaucrat?
3. How did he react to the news of the stranger about his illness?
4. Compare and contrast the reaction of his co-workers and his family to his illness.

5. Describe and discuss the moment in time with Ms. Odigiri that changed his life.
6. Why is it that Mr. Watanabe dies a contented man?
7. Do you expect his family or co-workers to understand his contentment? Explain.

Sophocles, *Philoktetes*

1. Why was Philoktetes deserted on Lemnos?
2. Who was he?
3. Describe Philoktetes' psychological and physical suffering.
4. What sacrifice does Neoptolemus make in order to gain Philoktetes' trust?
5. Why does Philoktetes refuse Neoptolemus' help near the end of the play?
6. Describe the ways in which Neoptolemus is able to be of assistance to Philoktetes.
7. What lies behind Odysseus' motive for deception?

Tolstoi, *The Death of Ivan Ilych*

1. Describe Ivan as a young man.
2. Describe Praskovya as a young woman.
3. Discuss their early years of marriage concentrating on the ways in which they related to one another.
4. Compare and contrast these early years with those during which so many of their children died and Ivan first became ill.
5. Ivan and Praskovya experienced his last illness in different ways. What are they and how do these personal reactions affect the other?
6. How did their children react to his illness?
7. Compare and contrast the reactions of Ivan's law colleagues and those of his doctors. How did these reactions affect Ivan?

8. Discuss Ivan's moral suffering.

9. Why didn't Ivan feel physical pain the last hours of his life?

Cather, "Paul's Case"

1. Describe Paul's way of getting through school days and home life.
2. What were his greatest fears and pleasures?
3. What did his flourishing fantasy life accomplish?
4. Why, exactly, did he run away to New York?
5. What occurred there that ultimately destroyed his hope?
6. Explain why it is that Paul succumbed to suicide.

Bernanos, *Mouchette*

1. Did Mouchette's poverty cause her despair?
2. How did she reason out solutions to problems?
3. Explain why it is exactly that the women in her community contributed to her untimely death.
4. How did Mouchette relate to her mother and father? Her brothers?
5. Why is it that she could not reveal what Arséne did to her?
6. What were the causes of the dissolution of her will?

Mouchette and Paul

1. Compare and contrast Paul and Mouchette's home and school life.
2. Compare and contrast their day dreaming and lying, and its purpose.
3. Compare and contrast their inner thoughts, ways of reasoning, of making decisions.
4. Compare and contrast the last hours of their lives in relation to their states of emotion, memory, and will.

5. Compare and contrast their loss of self-realization and its influence on their suicides.

Mason, *Gilgamesh*

1. Who was Gilgamesh? Why was he a tyrant?
2. Who was Enkidu? Why was he so innocent?
3. How do the two men become friends? Why is their friendship important to each?
4. What are the manifestations of Gilgamesh's grief?
5. How does friendship and loss humanize the tyrant king?
6. What journey does Gilgamesh undertake? Why is grief his only companion?
7. What events in this verse narrative tell us that there is no time limit to grief, but rather that it is a journey?

Bibliography

Bernanos, Georges. *Mouchette*. Translated from the French *Nouvelle histoire de Mouchette* by J. C. Whitehouse, 1966. New York: Holt, Rinehart, and Winston.

Campbell, Lewis. *Sophocles*, 1880. New York: Appleton.

Cather, Willa. "Paul's Case" in *Great Short Stories of Willa Cather*, 1989. New York: Harper and Row.

Gilgamesh: A retelling. Translated by Herbert Mason, 1972. New York: New American Library.

Kurosawa, Akira. *Ikiru*. A film script in Classic Film Scripts. English translation by Kurosawa Productions, 1968. Original Japanese language film entitled *Ikiru*, 1952 by Toho/Kurosawa Productions. Great Britain: Lorrimer Publishing.

Sophokles. *Philoktetes*, translated by Gregory McNamee, 1986. Port Townsend: Copper Canyon Press.

Tolstoi, Leo. *The Death of Ivan Ilych*, translated by Aylmer Maude, 1960. New York: New American Library.

Young-Mason, Jeanine. "Gilgamesh: A Consolation for Loss" in "Nursing and the Arts," *Clinical Nurse Specialist*, 1991: Vol. 5(2), p. 121–122.

_____ . "Two Stories of Adolescent Suicide" in "Nursing and the Arts" *Clinical Nurse Specialist*, 1992: Vol. 6(1), p. 151–152.

_____ . "Tolstoi's *The Death of Ivan Ilych:* A Source for Understanding Compassion." *Clinical Nurse Specialist,* 1988: Vol. 2(4), p. 180–183.

_____ . "Literature as a Mirror to Compassion." *Journal of Professional Nursing,* 1988: Vol. 4(4), p. 299–301.

_____ . "Visual Clues to Emotional States: Rodin's 'Burghers of Calais' " *Journal of Professional Nursing.* (Photographs by author). September/October, 1990: Vol. 6(5), p. 289–299.

_____ . "Kurosawa's *Ikiru:* A Compelling Film for the Study of Compassion." *Möbius.* 1987: Vol. (3), p. 49–52.

Appendix A

FURTHER SELECTIONS

Following is a selection of works of art, film, and fiction which have also been studied in the same fashion as the works in this text. They, too, have an inherent dialectic which has the ability to stimulate the student's sense of argument and analogy to everyday life and its contentions, oppositions, and polarizations. The works are arranged according to the major themes of: beginning nursing practice; character studies; and the roots of poverty and disease.

Beginning a Nursing Practice:

Joseph Conrad. *The Secret Sharer*, 1982. New York: Bantum.

Georges Bernanos. *The Diary of a Country Priest*, 1989. New York: Carroll & Graf Publishers, Inc.

Akira Kurosawa. *Akahige (Red Beard)*, 1965. Toho/Kurosawa Productions. Japan Black/White/185 minutes. Japanese language with English subtitles. May be rented or purchased in VHS format or rented as a 16mm film from *Facets Multimedia*, 1517 West Fullerton Ave., Chicago, Illinois 60614. Tel. (800) 331-6197.

Character Sketches:

Gustave Flaubert. *Madame Bovary*, 1972. Translated by Lowell Bair. New York: Bantum.

Albert Camus. *The Stranger*, 1988. Translated by Matthew Ward. New York: Random House.

Fyodor Dostoevki. *Notes from the Underground*, 1974. Translated by Mirra Ginsburg. New York: Bantum.

James Joyce. *Dubliners*, 1976. New York: Penguin.

Franz Kafka. *Metamorphosis*. In *Selected Short Stories of Franz Kafka* Translated by Willa and Edwin Muir, 1952. New York: Modern Library.

Herman Melville. "Billy Budd," "Bartleby" & "Benito Cereno" in *Billy Budd & Other Stories*, 1988. New York: Penguin.

Willa Cather. *Great Short Stories of Willa Cather*, 1989. New York: Harper & Row.

Flannery O'Conner. *The Complete Stories*, 1979. New York: Farrar, Straus & Giroux.

The Roots of Poverty and Disease:

George Orwell. *The Road to Wigan Pier*, 1958. New York: Harcourt Brace Jovanovich.

George Orwell. "How the Poor Die," in *The Orwell Reader*, 1956. New York: Harcourt, Brace and World.

Monsieur Vincent. French language with English subtitles. May be purchased on VHS Video Tape from *Foothill Video*, 7730 Foothill Blvd., Tujunga, CA 91042. Tel. (818) 353-8591.

Sister Kenny. Produced by Dudley Nichols, RKO Pictures, Inc., 1946. Turner Entertainment Company.

Appendix B

SOURCE NOTES TO RODIN, "THE BURGHERS OF CALAIS"

1. Froissart, J.: *Chronicles.* Translated and edited by Geoffrey Bererton. Middlesex, England: Harmondsworth, 1968, pp. 97–110.

2. McNamara, M.: *Rodin's "Burghers of Calais."* Stanford, CA: Stanford University, 1983, pp. 76–147, 181–187, 221, 275 (doctoral dissertation)

3. Anonymous: *Cloud of Unknowing.* Translated by Wolters, C. Great Britain, 1961, pp. 137–138.

4. Rodin, A.: *Art: Conversations with Paul Gsell.* Translated by de Caso, J. & Sanders, P. B. Berkeley: University of California Press, 1984, pp. 9–13, 37, 38, 84. In Rodin A: L'Art: Réunis par Paul Gsell. Paris, France: Grasset, 1911.

5. Lampert, C.: *Rodin: Sculpture and Drawings,* Arts Council of Great Britain. Musée Rodin and Spadem. New Haven, CT: Yale University Press, 1987, pp. 103–115.

6. Rilke, R. N.: *Rodin.* Translated by Firmage, R. Salt Lake City, UT: Peregrine, 1982, pp. 59, 60, 62.

7. Champignuelle, B.: *Rodin.* Translated by Brownjohn, J. M. New York: Oxford University Press, 1967, pp. 11, 87–91.

8. Tancock, J. L.: *The Sculpture of Auguste Rodin.* Philadelphia: Philadelphia Museum of Art & Godine Press, 1976, pp. 396, 397.